Freedom from PCOS

3 Proven Steps to Naturally Overcome Polycystic Ovarian Syndrome and Insulin Resistance

Katie Humphrey

Contents

Foreword

During my 25 years of developing wellness programs for people who are weight loss resistant, I have identified and found ways to overcome the biggest obstacles to living well and loving life.

When I read Katie Humphrey's book, I was reminded of so many women that I've met who struggle with Polycystic Ovarian Syndrome. These women not only deal with the horrific side effects of the syndrome, but are also deeply weight loss resistant. In working with such women, I have observed their heartbreak, and I have always searched for the best options to meet their specific needs.

Freedom from PCOS provides fresh insight and practical steps toward eliminating the symptoms of PCOS and achieving a healthful and balanced life. I find it to be a timely rescue for women who have been misunderstood and discouraged by the both the medical and nutrition communities.

Katie's book is born from her personal experience with PCOS but is supported by solid research. She writes with a voice of compassion and offers simple advice that yields powerful results. You will find encouragement, community and a strategy for living well within these pages. If you are a woman burdened by PCOS, I implore you to read and apply the message of this book.

JJ Virgin, PhD, CNS, Author of *Six Weeks to Sleeveless and Sexy*

Introduction

Why I Wrote this Book

Polycystic Ovarian Syndrome. The first time I heard this term I was 24 and hadn't had a menstrual period in four months. I wasn't pregnant and I wasn't taking birth control pills. I had gained over 25 pounds in just three months, and no one, not even me, knew why. Was I a secret binge eater? No, but no amount of greasy potato chips or sweet chocolate could satiate me or quiet the raging cravings that overcame me each and every day. Was I pre-menopausal? That was a possibility; though I was young for this type of diagnosis. Doctors and friends speculated that I was prematurely going through "the change." I had night sweats, hot flashes, crazy mood swings and irritability. My digestion got to the point where it simply quit working, and there was not a laxative on the market that could ease my discomfort.

Even with these challenges, I never stopped fighting, pushing, or searching to know the cause of my suffering. I felt alone, misunderstood, and pathetic. The day I heard my doctor speak my true condition (PCOS), I felt immediate panic instead of relief. I thought I would come to a place where I would find my answer and feel liberated, but it wasn't the case. PCOS? What was that? What could anyone do to help me? I was brushed off by my doctor, which forced me on a journey that brought me to where I am today.

I am 30 pounds lighter and free as can be. My menstrual cycle functions normally. I don't live under the bondage of PMS, and I certainly don't sweat during the day or at night like I used to. I run my own company, and I do what I love: I help women globally by informing them of the choices they have when living with a condition like PCOS. I let them know that I, too, have gone through the nightmare of not knowing what was wrong with my body; the empty place where you feel alone, worthless and defeated. So it is now my mission to inform, motivate and empower women with PCOS to take control over their condition naturally, just like I did.

In this book you will find the information you have been looking for if you want to control and overcome PCOS naturally, without any type of synthetic medication. Even though I don't personally know you yet, I love you just the same. I love you because we are kindred spirits, brought together by a terrifying condition, but united through the possibility of natural relief from our condition. I have done my best to give you the "short cuts" to changing the way your body currently operates with PCOS. This book will give you the tools and resources to replicate the steps I took to naturally overcome PCOS. But remember, no matter what you read in this book, the first change that must take place for you to create any type of success in your health is the change in your mindset. Up until now, you may have been engulfed in negativity and fear. For any change to take place, you must first begin with your own mental attitude. I completely transformed my body and health without the use of any unnatural method, but most importantly, I created a mindset of love, gratitude and abundance. This has kept me going in times of hardship and has allowed me to persevere through obstacles. Create this place of love and appreciation within yourself first, and you will be motivated to apply what you learn in this book, unyielding in your approach and joyful in your successes and temporary defeats. A positive mental attitude is my biggest victory in overcoming PCOS, and I had to create it before I succeeded; in fact, I had to create it to succeed! Do this for yourself, and you will be successful in anything you do. I look forward to hearing about the amazing changes you make in your health, and I wish you love and blessings on the journey you're about to take.

Chapter 1

The Facts, Jack

PCOS (Polycystic Ovarian Syndrome) is a serious endocrine disorder that affects one in ten women, according to the U.S. Department of Health and Human Services. PCOS can occur in females as young as eleven, although many women are not diagnosed with the condition until they reach childbearing age.

Some of the symptoms women with PCOS may experience include:

- Unexplained or uncontrollable weight gain
- Obesity
- Insulin resistance
- Type 2 diabetes
- High blood pressure
- Male-patterned baldness
- Acne
- Irregular and absent menstrual periods
- Ovarian cysts
- Infertility

Some women see very few of these symptoms and others experience an extreme amount. Don't go blaming mom just yet. There are several theories as to the origin of PCOS aside from genetics. The true cause is still unknown.

Unfortunately, doctors are only familiar with a few treatment options for PCOS. The first and most common treatment is birth control medication. Various types of birth control are used to regulate menstrual periods and balance hormonal levels. This is what I was given at the age of 18 and is still what doctors try to prescribe me when learning I have PCOS. The second treatment option is some type of Diabetic medication, which is used to control insulin levels. Anti-androgen prescriptions are used to combat hair loss and acne. For women wanting to conceive children, there are fertility medications that increase the chance of pregnancy.[1]

Isn't it great? We women with PCOS can "pop a pill or slap a patch on our bottoms" for every problem we face. Taking prescription medications can control symptoms and life can go back to normal. All of the problems stemming from your irregular or absent menstrual cycle—the male patterned baldness, crazy hair growth in all the wrong places, mood swings, cravings, weight gain, obesity, exhaustion and infertility – can be masked with a few man-made products. After all, if you have PCOS, you know what it is like to live this nightmare. All of this medication can solve your problems, right?

I was diagnosed with PCOS in 2007, and I decided that my life would not be consumed with medications, prescription pills, or anything unnatural as a means to control my condition. If you would like to live a life free from the devastating effects of PCOS, without the use of synthetic medication, read on, my friend, because there is hope for you.

Let's Sum It Up:

- PCOS (Polycystic Ovarian Syndrome) occurs in 1 in 10 women.
- Symptoms include an array of reproductive, hormonal and physiological problems.
- Researchers are unsure of the cause of PCOS.
- Many doctors are only familiar with synthetic medication options to treat PCOS.
- There are natural, alternative options to treat PCOS.

Chapter 2

My Personal Journey

From the time I hit puberty, I experienced serious hormonal imbalance. I'm talking about extreme symptoms that seemed to come from nowhere, making my already-awkward teen years an unforgettable nightmare. My menstrual cycles were never regular; I didn't even get a menstrual period until I was almost 15 years old. While normal girls were getting their menstrual periods around 12 and 13, I was embarrassed at the fact that I hadn't gotten mine. When I finally did get my first period, there were times when 3 months would go by before I would get another one. When it came, I would succumb to horrible bouts of anger and irritability. I would sort of "target" specific people, like my brother, on which to unleash my fury. My mom thought I was "possessed" by an evil spirit every time I would get my period because of the rage I exhibited.

If my menstrual cycle weren't coming in 3 month intervals, I would get it two weeks apart. The pain I felt with intense menstrual cramps and achiness in my abdomen and lower back was excruciating. I truly thought that other girls were going through the same thing I was, but that wasn't the case. I also had really bad acne on my face, and I would crave greasy, junk foods and sugary sweets. I remember hating all of my school pictures because of my bad complexion. Needless to say, I felt out of control and hopeless as a teenager. I was awkward and out of place because of my symptoms. I couldn't stand the way I was. I didn't know what was wrong with me.

By the time I was 18, my mom urged me to see an OB/GYN to discuss my options in balancing my hormonal levels. I think she was at her wits end more than I was. I know she felt sorry for me, but she didn't really know how to help me at the time. The doctor prescribed me birth control pills to control my moods and regulate my menstrual cycles. We had to experiment with 3 different types of oral contraceptives before we found one that agreed with my body. I remember putting a "patch" on my butt, and other various places, only to gain 15 pounds in 4 weeks because the hormones were too strong for my body. I was taking birth control pills for about two years before my symptoms started to calm down.

For a short time, I experienced normalcy from taking birth control. This quickly changed when I entered college and developed an unhealthy lifestyle. By the time I was in my sophomore year in college, I had gained twenty pounds and suffered from a variety of hormonal issues including night sweats, irritability, sugar/alcohol/carbohydrate cravings, and PMS. Due to my college lifestyle, it was as if my body was desensitized to the birth control pills. Because of this, I started taking natural supplements here-and-there to control my other symptoms.

It was finally clear to me that birth control was not the answer to restoring my health. I was tired of the excess weight and dealing with symptoms common in menopausal women. In 2007, I did what I thought was the brave thing and stopped taking birth control pills altogether. I was afraid that these synthetic hormones would do long-term damage to my body. I had heard too many rumors about women who suffered from a stroke, heart condition, or other type of serious disease, all of which were possibly linked to birth control pills. I thought, *I can't stay on these pills forever!* I doubted I would even notice a difference if I stopped taking them.

Unfortunately, at the time, going off birth control seemed to awaken a beast within me that I did not know existed. As soon as I stopped taking birth control, I immediately ceased to have a menstrual cycle and started to put on weight! A few pounds crept up within a month, though I didn't think much of it at first. I soon noticed, however, that my appetite for sweets and carbohydrates was insatiable. As time went on, my energy levels began to drop, and I constantly felt fatigued.

Within two months I had gained 20 pounds, and by Christmas I had gained a total of 30 pounds. I remember sitting on my bedroom floor, as I attempted to find something to where for my mother's Christmas Eve party, sobbing. None of my clothes fit, and the pants I bought the previous month, which were 2 sizes bigger than my usual size, no longer fit. They were super tight, and it was devastating. I could not understand what was wrong with me. Was I a big, fat pig who could not quit eating? What had I done to put on so much weight, and why wasn't it coming off?

I tried to control my weight with strict eating habits and exercise. Although I thought I was already a pretty healthy eater, I felt I was obviously doing something wrong. I read every book I could get my hands on about nutrition, dieting, and weight loss. And though I had been exercising regularly for years, I felt I needed to step it up and work harder. I started exercising twice a day, sometimes 6 days a week! Big mistake. I would later learn that too much exercise can be counterproductive for women with PCOS.

I could not lose the weight no matter what I tried. Desperate for answers, I saw my regular MD the following month. She decided to do some blood tests, checking my hormone, thyroid, and blood sugar levels. Everything came back normal. I remember getting the call from my nurse practitioner who quickly said, "Everything is fine. Your tests were normal."

"Wait..." I replied. "What do you mean everything is normal? Can you please send me my test results? I don't understand!" The Nurse Practitioner shrugged me off, so I went to my doctor's office and got a copy of the results. I was annoyed and hurt that my doctor's office didn't seem to care that there was something really wrong with me. It made me feel isolated and alone that no one could understand what I was going through. I knew I wasn't crazy.

Refusing to accept my doctor's final diagnosis, I made an appointment to see an endocrinologist. After undergoing more blood work and explaining my health history in full detail, I was sure he would be the one to solve all of my problems. My blood work came back normal, but my testosterone levels were slightly elevated. The endocrinologist wrote a prescription for me to have a routine sonogram performed on my lower abdomen to see if I had any ovarian cysts. The test came back negative.

Freedom from PCOS

After everything he heard from me and witnessed on my tests, the doctor muttered something about "PCOS" or Polycystic Ovarian Syndrome, but told me I was healthy and within a normal weight range. He scribbled "PCOS" on my chart as the final diagnosis, but didn't explain anything about the condition.

"I'm sorry," I exclaimed, "but are you telling me that I'm perfectly healthy and that I should just leave?!" He explained that since he was an endocrinologist that I would have to see my OB/GYN to discuss my options for PCOS. Needless to say, I was completely frustrated at his response. I felt disappointed that my path had taken this detour. I truly expected to find a solution, but was turned away only to continue my search. What was PCOS? What is this disorder that has caused me so much pain and frustration? I decided to do my own due diligence to truly understand this condition.

When I did my own research on PCOS, I discovered that elevated testosterone levels were causing my acne, irregular menstrual periods and moodiness. I was also suffering from insulin resistance and hypoglycemia. My cells were not being receptive to the insulin produced in my body, thereby causing the sugar and carbohydrate cravings as well as the weight gain and body fat storage. My adrenal and pituitary glands were not functioning properly, causing major fatigue while disrupting the normal hormonal balance within my body.

I finally made an appointment to see a "natural" OBGYN who was known to do natural hormone therapy as opposed to synthetic medication prescriptions. "Unfortunately," she told me, after reviewing my symptoms and blood work results, "the only treatment to counter the effects of Polycystic Ovarian Syndrome is birth control pills. I'll also give you something to stabilize your insulin levels."

She proceeded to tell me that I would have to be on birth control until I hit menopause, breaking every 5 years for 6 months to give my body a rest from the medication. If I ever wanted children, I would have to take fertility medications, and I would have to conceive as soon as possible. *I just got married a month ago*, I thought, *I'm not even ready for kids yet!* I immediately left the building, saying, "thanks, but no thanks." *Sure*, I thought sarcastically, *I'll just accept my weight gain, along with everything else I'm experiencing, and look forward to a catastrophic wave of side effects as I go off of birth control every several years!*

I got into my car and turned on the engine. "You've got to be kidding me!" I yelped as I began to sob. I had held in my pain for so long and now it was all coming out all at once in a downpour of tears. I called my husband and told him it was over. I had found my answer, and it was the same "answer" I had rebelled against almost 11 months earlier. As I regained composure, I realized that I had nowhere else to turn. No one else was going to solve my problem, so it was time to take matters into my own hands.

I began to do a tremendous amount of research on PCOS, reading every bit of information I could find. Miraculously, while researching PCOS on the internet, I found a company that offered all natural supplements as part of a protocol to combat PCOS and insulin resistance. I researched the ingredients as well as the company as a whole. I even shared the information with my mom, who owns an online store that specializes in organic and natural supplements. She reviewed the ingredients and gave the company her approval. My husband and I decided that it was best to try their trial program for at least six months. I figured that I had nothing to lose at this point. If this company's product didn't do as it promised, I could get my money back and move on. I had to try, though; I was willing to do whatever it took to find a natural solution.

Redemption!

Within 6 weeks I had lost 10 pounds and gained my energy back. I specifically remember the weight being gone during the time of my wedding reception. The dress I had bought and had altered was falling down at the reception! It was a fantastic, but an embarrassing problem to have. My sweet cravings were kept to a minimum. With my cravings minimized, I was able to make conscious, healthy food choices. If I did not make it clear before, my sugar, carbohydrate and alcohol cravings were previously uncontrollable and insatiable! It was a miracle to not be constantly thinking about and craving unhealthy foods.

Two months later, 1 had lost another 5 pounds. I began to exercise in a whole new way. I learned that women with PCOS need to exercise differently than men, especially if we want to balance our bodies naturally. I also started to eat healthily about 80% of the time, while having the occasional treat 20% of the time. All the while, my night sweats and hot flashes had completely disappeared. This was the first time these symptoms had vanished since puberty. My digestion was also functioning at an optimal level. I had never in my life experienced good digestion. This was such a blessing!

By February 2009, 6 months after starting the supplement program, I had lost all the weight and was in better shape than before I gained all the weight. I felt free and empowered! I decided to become a personal trainer and supportive life coach to teach other women how to live healthier, happier lives doing exactly what I will share in this book.

My body now has the ability to naturally regulate my hormones. Since then I have had little, if any, side effects from my monthly cycle. I no longer experience crazy mood swings and I rarely get menstrual cramps. The skin on my face is clear and my energy is high throughout the day.

Deciding to quit taking birth control pills is the best decision I have ever made. By doing my own research into PCOS and not accepting the diagnoses and options recommended by various doctors, I have been able to successfully control PCOS and insulin resistance naturally. It is now my hope and mission in life to help other women do the same.

Let's Sum It Up:
- I have suffered from the effects of PCOS since puberty.
- I started taking birth control pills at the age of 18.
- Five years later I quit taking birth control pills "cold turkey" to be free of synthetic medications.

- Going off of birth control pills was the only way I would have known about my condition.
- I found a reputable company whose natural supplements combat and possibly reverse the symptoms associated with PCOS.
- Within 6 months on the natural supplements, I was mostly symptom-free and got in great physical shape.
- My success motivated me to help other women achieve similar results.
- I now empower women to use holistic methods to achieve true freedom from PCOS.

Chapter 3

My Problem, Your Solution

When I look back, I am grateful to have gone through my experience with PCOS and insulin resistance. However, before I discovered effective supplements – combined with lifestyle changes – for PCOS, there was a time I wished I had stayed on birth control. Before I knew there was a solution, I would sometimes give up hope, thinking there was no "light at the end of the tunnel." Think of a time when you were halfway on a long, hard journey and giving up and turning around crossed your mind. You sensed there was an answer to your problem, but you were not completely sure of it. What if an "answer" presented itself, but it didn't feel right? What if everyone was telling you how to "fix" your problem but you sincerely believed they were mistaken? When life seemed unbearable and I felt fat and very much like a failure, I pushed forward. I knew the right answer was out there somewhere; a solution that could remedy my condition. Even though fear would sometimes creep in, something inside me kept pushing and asking me to stand strong and keep fighting until it was over.

Finding the right combination to combat PCOS and insulin resistance took me an extremely long time. There were times when I was the only one believing in my mission to find a "natural" answer, but victory was sweet when I found it. Being ignorant, naïve, or remaining in denial about your condition is no way to live. Sooner or later you will see the long-term effects of PCOS impact your body and life. My journey may have been challenging at times, but the experience allowed me to triumph over my condition, become a life coach for women, and create my own company and its programs. This book, in and of itself, would have never come to be had I not gone through what I did. I believe that I had to undergo this terrible experience in my life so I could help other women like you. My goal is to let as many women with PCOS and insulin resistance know that there is hope and that solutions do exist. This is an important and powerful message for me to deliver because I wish someone would have had a similar message when I needed answers.

There are things you can do to get your condition under control and possibly reverse it. I know you will find everything in this book to be something you can implement easily into your life. I have taken the time to provide you with a step-by-step process of exactly what I did to reverse my condition. You are going to receive answers to losing weight effectively and permanently; controlling those insatiable cravings, increasing energy levels, regulating your menstrual cycle and reducing symptoms associated with your monthly cycle. You will also be able to control and reduce acne and hair loss and feel in control of your diet and condition. If I did it, so can you! So, please, take the time and read through everything. You can start incorporating the steps as you read them or after you are done reading everything. Please make sure you thoroughly cover everything. Most likely I will have answered many of your questions regarding this condition. So sit back, read, and relax knowing there is proven success to combating PCOS and insulin resistance. You are finally going to be in control. The answers are here!

My struggle pushed me to find answers, which are now your simple solution. The dark time in my life has given me a new appreciation of my current life, free of PCOS. Take the time to read through the entire book, and I look forward to hearing about your results and your progress. Remember, I am here for you, I love you and I know you can do it.

Let's Sum It Up:

- Had I not gone through my struggle with PCOS and insulin resistance, I would not have come to the place in my life today.

- My problem is your solution. I hope my story inspires you to make healthy changes so that you, too, can be free from the bonds of PCOS.

Chapter 4

PCOS and its Long-term Effects

Among the research material I found were devastating facts for women with PCOS. According to the U.S. Department of Health and Human Services, more than 50% of women with PCOS will have diabetes or pre-diabetes before the age of 40. This single fact absolutely blew me away. Notice the wording used: *more* than 50% of women with PCOS *will* have diabetes or pre-diabetes before 40. That means it is more than a potential problem; it's a fact! It's a guarantee that half of women like us will end up with either of these horrible conditions.[1]

This is not something you want in your life. I used to work at a company that sold medical supplies for men and women with diabetes. Most of the personal stories of our patients were disheartening. Diabetes is a serious condition that can lead to many health complications. Diabetics have to regularly monitor blood sugar levels and experience many problems with blood circulation and organ function, including liver, kidney, pancreas, and eye problems.[2] My Uncle Steve was a diabetic and died in his early sixties due to complications from his condition. The end of his life was spent in a nursing home as a double amputee, suffering and waiting for the sweet release of death. I know that sounds really morbid, but it was such a rough and terribly sad time for my family, especially my father, as we watched Steve endure his final days. If diabetes is already in your family history, you need to take more precaution and gain control over your health before it's too late.

Women with PCOS are also 4 to 7 times more likely to have a heart attack than women without PCOS. This condition can also cause high blood pressure and high cholesterol levels if left unchecked. High blood pressure and high cholesterol already lead to coronary heart disease which is a precursor for a heart attack. Heart disease is the number one killer in the United States, and it is a scary thought to think that we women with PCOS are *4* to *7* times more likely to develop it!

These can be extreme circumstances, but they are real nonetheless. Please feel free to check my sources for these facts, and do research for yourself. You will find further evidence of other major health complications for which women with PCOS and insulin resistance are at high risk. You will see that there are different cancers that we are more susceptible to, like endometrial cancer.[1] Sounds pleasant, no? If you have PCOS then you know it is no picnic dealing with the condition itself. Tack on diabetes, high blood pressure, cholesterol, and the risk of a heart attack, and you are a walking death sentence.

If you want to avoid any future health complications, it is recommended to get your condition under control as soon as possible.

Before you go running off to your doctor for a prescription, keep reading.

Control PCOS Naturally

I am happy to say that I have been off birth control pills, as well as any other type of synthetic medication, since 2007. I do not use medicine for colds, headaches, muscular cramps or anything else. I never take anything because I do not have to. I eat, exercise and take supplements that allow my body to naturally regulate its systems. I rarely get sick because my immune system has been dramatically strengthened, and I no longer suffer from serious P.M.S. because my hormones are balanced. On the rare occasion I come down with a cold or have a slight tension headache, I go to my acupuncturist and get the problem taken care of naturally. However, bacterial infections are a different story: medication may be *necessary* for bacterial infections. And please do not mistake me and think that you do not need to see your doctor if you have any type of sickness, illness, condition or disease. Quite the contrary; please *always* consult your doctor and decide which medication is absolutely necessary. If you have a cold, taking over-the-counter drugs to only mask symptoms is not always wise. **Your focus should be to heal the condition, not cover up symptoms.** Use discernment when taking medication prescribed by your doctor.

The point is that once all foreign, synthetic medication has left the body, it can naturally regulate, balance and heal itself. The reason I say "foreign," is because chemically altered drugs, as in almost every prescription and over the counter drug we know, are not something our bodies are used to or familiar with. When you take an aspirin, it may relieve the inflammation causing you pain, but you are not allowing your body to do *its* job. Our bodies have natural pain relievers and they

27

cannot be accessed when you take a pill that steps in and does it for you. What's worse is that if you have to take an aspirin all the time, you are not addressing the core issue as to why you are having pain in the first place. When I say things like this, I always have people respond with, "What if someone is constantly suffering from aches and pains?" If you have severe pain, then you would benefit from knowing that research has proven that different foods can reduce inflammation naturally. Usually people who are in the most pain are not eating a healthy diet or the right diet for their condition.

When you only put natural things in your body, you become acutely in tune with it. I refused to accept my OB/GYN's recommendation to "continue taking birth control until I hit menopause," because I believed there was a better, more natural way. When you take any type of medication, you are basically telling your body, "You cannot do the job properly." When I was taking birth control pills, I was telling my body that I could not regulate my hormonal system the way it needed to be regulated, so my body refused to have a menstrual period for twenty months after I quit taking the pills. Now I have a regular, five-day menstrual period without any of the cramps, headaches, or quirky digestion problems I used to experience. My menstrual periods are so subtle; if I am not tracking them they sneak up on me! The funny thing is, even on birth control, I suffered from serious P.M.S., even though the pills were supposed to reduce and/or control the symptoms associated with my menstrual cycles.

Again, consult your doctor before you decide to take or quit taking any type of prescribed medicine. Just remember, this is the one body you were given in the one life you will live. Treat it well and it will reward you.

Don't Assume it's PCOS

Please do not be the woman who reads about the symptoms associated with PCOS and self-diagnoses based on her findings. A formal diagnosis from a doctor is recommended and encouraged. I had a friend who read all of my information on PCOS and mistakenly thought she had the condition. When I urged her to seek a diagnosis from her doctor, she discovered that she had hypothyroidism. Many women with hypothyroidism mistakenly believe they have PCOS because the two conditions are very similar. In fact, I was sure I had hypothyroidism before I was diagnosed with PCOS.

If you are unsure of whether or not you have this condition, please make an appointment with your regular doctor or request to see an endocrinologist. I recommend seeing an endocrinologist because most doctors may not be familiar with the formal diagnosis of PCOS or insulin resistance.

Once you see your doctor, explain that you believe you suffer from Polycystic Ovarian Syndrome and be ready to describe, in detail, the symptoms you have experienced from as far back as you can remember (this may be puberty for some). Also be sure that your doctor prescribes specific blood work to be done; while there is no specific test to diagnose PCOS, ask to have your hormonal, specifically testosterone, insulin and fasting blood sugar levels checked. You can also request to have an abdominal sonogram to check for ovarian cysts.

Be warned: if your doctor diagnoses you with PCOS and/or insulin resistance, he or she will most likely recommend you be put on birth control pills and possibly other medications to help regulate insulin. As mentioned before, I recommend you go the natural route as described in this book. It is your body; do what you think is right. Taking birth control and other medications may seem like the easy way out, but you are setting yourself up for failure. You will never gain true control over your body or your condition if you put unnatural substances in it. Fortunately, after learning about my "Triple Threat" approach to PCOS, you will not look twice at birth control pills or any other prescription pill.

Let's Sum It Up:
- More than 50% of women with PCOS will have pre-diabetes or diabetes before the age of 40.
- Women with PCOS are 4 to 7 times more likely to have a heart attack than women without the condition.
- Women with PCOS are at a higher risk for endometrial cancer.
- Your focus should be on healing the condition, not masking symptoms (birth control masks PCOS symptoms, it does not heal the core issue)
- Talk to your doctor before deciding to take or quit taking any medication
- Don't think you have PCOS just because you identify with some of the symptoms; get a formal diagnosis.

- There is no one test that doctors use to diagnose PCOS, though you should request specific blood work to check your hormone, insulin and fasting blood sugar levels.
- Your doctor should also request an abdominal sonogram to check for ovarian cysts.
- Know that you will have to inevitably make a choice as to how you want to treat PCOS.

Chapter 5

My Triple Threat Approach to Overcome PCOS

My "Triple Threat" approach to PCOS and insulin resistance will not only give you a healthy, trim body, but it will also make you feel naturally energized and in control. It sounds so simple that you are going to think I am crazy for recommending it. But it works and nothing else out there has worked for me. It took me more than two years to find the perfect combination of exercising, eating the right foods, and taking specific supplements (see Figure 1). Once I did, it took less than 8 months for me to completely transform my body and overcome PCOS. I know that once you implement it, you will see great results, too.

Exercise, proper nutrition and specific nutraceuticals gave me the edge I needed to get back the thin, energetic, regulated, balanced body I had not seen for years. These three strategies, in a specific combination, will help you yield the results you want. And if you think you have already tried one of these approaches and it did not work, hang on. I am going to show you exactly what I did and how it can help you.

The beautiful part about the Triple Threat approach is that it *is* so simple; it is crazy to think you could have been doing any one of these things all along.

This is not about being extreme – quite the opposite. Take everything at your own level. You will not have to exercise every day. You will not have to cut out any food groups, nor will you have to give up dessert.

Figure 1

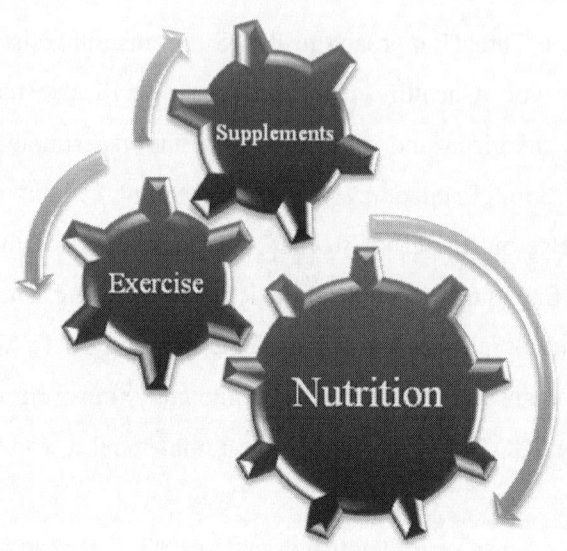

Let's Sum It Up:

- My Triple Threat approach to combat and possibly reverse PCOS and insulin resistance includes exercise, eating right and taking nutraceuticals.

- This simple approach, when done as instructed, can help you achieve the results you were unable to get through any other means.

Chapter 6

Exercise Specifically for PCOS

Exercise is the first part of the Triple Threat approach to overcome PCOS. Exercise has positive effects on the body's response to insulin, and it is the easiest strategy to implement.[3] Our bodies were made to move around, not sit on our rear ends all day. It may seem like hard work in the beginning, but after a while you will find exercise a fun, necessary part of your daily routine.

I heard a podcast the other day in which the gentleman noted that exercise is tough work. "Even physically advanced men and women feel that exercise is tough conditioning," said the host. Nonsense! I find exercise to be easy, enjoyable and downright exciting. To be able to move around without getting out of breath, and to feel your body become stronger, leaner, and more flexible, is as exhilarating as it sounds.

I also recommend exercise first because, as I tell all of the clients I coach, even if the weight isn't coming off just yet does *not* mean you are working in vain. The body is a beautiful creation. It will quietly retain lean muscle, become better conditioned, and improve in every area while you are figuring out other changes that need to be made to see results.

Exercise burns calories, sheds fat, and naturally reduces cholesterol, high blood pressure, the risk of heart disease, diabetes, and other serious health conditions.[4] In the beginning it can be tedious, but once you are used to it, usually within a month, you will feel fresh and revitalized. Exercising also becomes addictive. You will notice that once you have established an exercise habit, you will feel gross or even guilty if skip a session. Do not worry though: it is a good addiction to have. It is a shame to waste a body that has the ability to move around. Use your body to exercise and you will reap the sweet benefits it has to offer. There are several types of exercises I recommend but I will show you the ones to implement that will make the biggest difference. Cardiovascular exercise and strength training are the two main types of exercises on which I will focus.

Let's Sum It Up:
- Exercise increases the body's response to insulin being produced.
- It can be fun, easy and exciting.
- Exercise burns calories, increases energy and reduces the risk of serious health conditions.
- There are two types of exercise we will focus on: cardio and strength training.

Chapter 7

Two Types of Cardio

Cardiovascular, commonly known as cardio, exercise not only burns calories and improves the condition of your heart, lungs and organs, but it also improves your body's sensitivity to insulin. This is especially important in women with insulin resistance. You want your body to respond to the insulin being produced, and cardio is one way to increase this response.

There are two types of cardio that you should be performing: Steady-state and intervals.

Cardio Type #1: Steady-State

Steady-state cardio is exactly what it sounds like. You choose a form of cardio (it could be walking, biking, swimming, jogging, etc) and perform it for a certain amount of time at the *same* pace the entire time. For instance, if you start walking outside or on a treadmill, increase your pace until you feel as if it is moderately challenging while still comfortable, and stay at this pace the duration of the exercise.

It really does not matter what form of exercise you choose, but

Two Types of Cardio

I must say that it helps to switch it up once in a while. If you like rollerblading, start doing it 1 to 2 times a week, and in a few months do something new. Take up cycling or swimming for a change. Your may reach a point where it becomes accustomed to a specific type of exercise and halts weight loss. This is called hitting a plateau. You will find this to be true in many aspects of living a healthy life. That's why taking a break from exercise for a few days can have a positive impact on your body. The more you make exercise a lifetime habit, the more you will need to change around your routine. Be encouraged by the change. Trying new exercises every few months (or few weeks) can freshen up your routine, making it something new to look forward to.

Perform steady-state cardio 1 to 2 times a week for as long as you can up to 60 minutes. Start out by doing something for 10 to 15 minutes a day and work your way up to longer sessions. I personally walk or ride my home recumbent bike for about 20 to 45 minutes, depending on how much time and energy I have. Nothing is too short. If you can only do it for 10 minutes, do it. Everything is cumulative and it adds up quickly. Let's say that you only have time to go walking 10 minutes a day, even if it is 5 minutes in the morning and 5 minutes in the evening. After doing this for 5 days, you have walked between 2 to 3 miles. Within a month you will have walked 8 to 12 miles. Not bad for someone who does not have time to exercise. Any amount of steady-state cardio counts and doing it in short intervals will motivate you to do more.

Choose the type of cardio that seems the easiest or most fun to you (walking and riding my bike are my personal favorites), and start doing it today. Be encouraged to know that if you walk down the block and back, you have done *something*! Anything counts as long as you give it your best shot.

Let's Sum It Up:

- Performing any type of exercise at a consistent pace is steady-state cardio.
- Change up your cardio selection every few months.
- Perform steady-state cardio 1 or 2 times a week for 10 to 60 minutes.
- Doing cardio in small spurts throughout the day can have a positive effect.

Cardio Type #2: Intervals

Cardio intervals are performed by doing any type of exercise in different interval periods. The object of the exercise is to increase the intensity through speed or resistance one minute and slowing down to recover the next minute. The increase in intensity and cool down is repeated throughout the exercise. This type of cardio can effectively burn fat in a short period of time. It's best for those who are strapped for time and want a quick, effective workout.

Cardio intervals are great for burning the maximum amount of calories. Performing intervals allows you to burn calories up to 48 hours after you exercise, as a result of post-exercise oxygen consumption (commonly referred to as "EPOC" in the fitness industry). EPOC is the state in which the body uses energy to recover and attempts to reinstate every system back to homeostatic condition.[5] This is excellent news for those of us who want to burn maximum calories for many hours after exercising. The "energy" used is calories burned and it only takes about 20 minutes of fast and slow intervals to achieve this. Just to be clear, *steady-state* cardio burns calories during the exercise and up to about 30 minutes after you are done exercising. On the other hand, as I just mentioned, cardio *intervals* burn calories up to 48 hours after exercising. I want you to understand the difference between the two. We need both types of cardio exercise, but *intervals* are more efficient at burning fat and calories.

Intervals can be performed indoors or outside, with or without cardio equipment. Whichever medium you choose to do the cardio intervals, you need to perform one minute of "exertion" and one to two minutes of "recovery." Exertion is equivalent to pushing yourself to the maximum possible condition. Increasing your speed or resistance while exercising can do this. For instance, if you prefer walking outdoors or on a treadmill, do the intervals by jogging, running or sprinting for the "exertion" portion and walking for the "recovery" portion. Likewise if you are on a recumbent or trail bicycle, increase speed or resistance for the "exertion" duration and slow pedal as you recover. Some women think they are doing these intervals properly, but on the "recovery" portion, they are not slowing down as much as they should. The recovery is meant to decrease your heart rate to the point where you feel at rest and at ease. There should be a significant difference in your heart rate during the exertion and as you recover.

Let's pretend you are on a treadmill performing intervals. Here's an example of how you could do it:

1 minute - moderate speed, get the heart rate up ("power walking" at 3.7 with 1% incline)

1 minute - exertion - go hard (sprint at 6.3 with 1% incline)

2 minutes - recovery - get the heart rate down (walk at 3.0, no incline)

1 minute - exertion - push harder than last time! (sprint at 6.5 with 2% incline)

2 minutes - recovery - slow down the heart rate (walk at 3.0, no incline)

1 minute - exertion - push even harder now! (sprint at 6.7, 2% incline)

2 minutes -recovery (walk at 3.0, no incline)

1 minute - exertion - push, push, push! (sprint at 7.0, 2% incline)

2 minutes - recovery (walk at 3.0, no incline)

1 minute - exertion - push, push, push! (sprint at 7.0, 3% incline)

2 minutes -recovery (walk at 3.0, no incline)

1 minute - exertion – push harder than ever before! (sprint at 7.5, no incline)

3 minutes - recovery (walk at 3.0, no incline)

(This is a 20 minute plan. Intervals should be done between 18 – 20 minutes for best results).

Keep up this momentum for at least 18 minutes. During the exertion push harder each and every time. You should be going harder and faster than the previous exertion. The object is to force the heart and lungs to work hard. However, be wary of pushing yourself too hard if you are a beginner. Ease into the exertion portion and see how your body responds. If you are doing a walk/run for your intervals, you may want to start out "power walking" instead of running for the exertion part.

The most important thing to remember is to listen to your body. Also be sure you consult your doctor before engaging in a new exercise program.

When you come to the recovery part of the exercise, focus on slowing your heart rate as much as possible. Do whatever it takes to slow your breathing. Notice how the recovery was the same speed in the example listed above. You can walk, swim, rollerblade or cycle as slow as you want when you recover. The recovery time is meant to restore a high percentage of the energy that is used to push you during the exertion intervals.[5] Use this time to also think relaxing thoughts, drink some water and draw slow breaths. During the recovery intervals, I usually pause my iPod and focus on recovering. Once I begin the next intense interval, I crank the music and power through!

Cardio intervals will revive you and seriously increase your energy levels. Once you make this exercise a habit, you will appreciate the surge of fresh, invigorating aliveness you will feel in such a short time. Try to do 1 to 2 days of intervals a week for 18 to 20 minutes, and you will see results in no time. I personally do about 1 to 2 days of intervals a week, depending on how much steady-state cardio I am doing.

Please don't put too much pressure on yourself with these cardio exercises. I want you to ease into an exercise program. Try both the steady-state and intervals and work your way up to a longer duration of exercise. When I first started exercising, I would walk my sister's dog for 20 minutes, twice a week. Even in that short time, I felt more energized and healthy. You can do this. Just take it one small step at a time.

Remember, only you can hold yourself back from gaining true freedom in your health. Don't make excuses. Thinking of every reason why you *can't* do something is just fear talking. You have nothing to lose, and you will *not* end up worse than you already are. *Believe in your ability to do these exercises.*

Let's Sum It Up:
- Cardio intervals are an essential part of a fat-burning exercise program.
- The intervals cause the body to burn calories up to 48 hours after you are finished exercising due to EPOC.
- Intervals can be performed doing any type of exercise.
- Do cardio intervals 1 to 2 times a week for 18 to 20 minutes.
- Monitor breathing and heart rate. Beginners should ease in to the exertion portion of the exercise.

Cardio Fine Points:
- Perform both types of cardio exercises a total of 2 to 4 days a week. Beginners do 1 day of steady-state and 1 day of Intervals; work your way up to 3 to 4 days a week total.
- If you do 1 day of steady-state, do intervals the other 2 or 3 days,

and vice-versa.

- Don't put too much pressure on yourself. Take small steps and try both types of cardio.

- Listen to your body and challenge yourself, taking necessary breaks.

- Talk to your doctor before beginning any type of exercise program.

Additional Tips:

- **If you have access to a gym:** Utilize the cardio equipment. Both types of cardio can be done on a treadmill, recumbent bike, elliptical, Stairmaster, etc. Spin classes are also a great (though challenging) way to do intervals.

- **No gym:** Go outdoors (weather permitting) and do cardio by walking, swimming, cycling, rollerblading, etc. using the principles discussed above.

- **No energy:** Lack of energy in women with PCOS can be a product of excess weight gain and/or fatigued adrenal glands. If you lack the energy to exercise, find a time in the day when you have even the slightest amount of energy and do as much as you can. Even 10 minutes of walking is better than being sedentary or stuffing your face at home. You may feel more energy in the morning, afternoon or in the evening. Do what is necessary to maneuver work and family responsibilities so you are able to exercise at some point in the day.

- **Moms:** If you have access to one, perform cardio with a jogging stroller outdoors. If not, or if you cannot leave the house, get creative and do cardio in your living room by walking in place for 1 minute then running in place or doing jumping jacks for 1 minute; repeat for about 20 minutes. Holding your child while walking in place can really make you sweat!

- **Working women:** Plan exercise around your work schedule. Bring a change of clothes and exercise during your lunch break or before or after work hours. If you prefer to workout at home, get creative with your cardio (see instructions for "Moms"). You can purchase used exercise equipment through many online sites like craigslist.com. My husband and I bought a brand new exercise bike on one of these sites for a steal. Browse the internet for used equipment if you feel more comfortable exercising at home.

Chapter 8

Lean and Trim with Strength Training

Strength training is the other type of exercise that is particularly essential to combat weight gain from PCOS. Strength training can include any type of exercise that targets and conditions lean muscle in the body. Weight lifting using free weights, resistance bands, weight machines, cables, or body weight is the quickest way to burn fat, lean down and prevent osteoporosis.[5] One of the reasons I originally became a personal trainer was to learn more of the science behind the fantastic results I was getting from strength training.

I learned that the more lean muscle added to the body, the smaller you will look. You will also burn more calories on a regular basis, and feel stronger. Most women are afraid of "building muscle" when deciding to participate in a strength training program. Let's just clear this myth up right now. Women do not normally get bulky or big when they put on muscle unless they use steroids and "body-builder" powders. In fact, once your body begins to burn off the fat on top of the muscle, you will actually look smaller and fitter than if you had no muscle.

It is a huge misconception that muscle and fat are the same thing. They are two completely separate entities. If you have big, jiggly arms, your arm fat is *not* going to turn into muscle of the same size, leaving you with Arnold Schwarzenegger arms. Quite the contrary, your arms will get smaller as the muscle burns off the fat. I have a client who started working with me because her granddaughter always commented on her "turkey triceps." The observation of this 4 year-old pushed her to start lifting free-weights to tone up her arms. To this day, she has beautiful arms – toned and lean – and it only took 12 weeks! Did I mention she is in her mid-fifties?

Think of it this way: A woman who has "abs of steel" has built muscle within her midsection. She has not just burned off fat from her abdominal muscles; she has actually put on muscle! If you are picturing the same woman I am, then you know that her abs do not look big or bulky; her waist is small, slim and sexy!

Adding lean muscle to the body also burns more calories at rest than any other exercise because muscle weighs more than fat.[5] The body has to use more energy moving around lean muscle on the body than it does jiggly fat. This means that if you add 5 pounds of lean muscle on your body, you will start burning a ton more calories every minute than you are now, even when you are sleeping. Not to mention, if you put on 5 pounds of muscle, you will lose much more in fat, so you will not gain weight. You will lose weight and look tighter and tinier. This is the big secret to losing weight permanently that so many women have embraced.

Smart women know that putting on lean muscle is work in the beginning, but once you build lean muscle, it becomes less and less work to maintain. A very close girlfriend of mine has worked hard to put on lean muscle, and she and I beam at the fact that we do not have to exercise as much as we used to. We also love the fact that we can get away with eating less-than-healthy foods every once in a while because the added lean muscle burns so many calories! Now, let me be clear: I am not disclosing this information so you have an excuse to pig out all the time. It just helps to know that your efforts of putting on lean muscle can counteract the effects of holiday desserts.

Lean muscle is not only essential to weight loss, it is also recommended by doctors to help reduce the risk of osteoporosis.[6] Adding strong, lean muscle to the body protects bones. After the age of 40, women lose about 6-8% of lean muscle every decade.[7] This not only puts us at high risk for osteoporosis, it also means that we are burning fewer calories every year. No wonder women find it hard to lose weight as they get older! If women maintain regular exercise, especially in strength training, weight loss is a cinch. And I don't want to hear any griping about this. I have heard women tell me, "It isn't easy to put on muscle after the age of 40." Nonsense! One of my best clients just turned fifty, and she is mostly muscle. When she is out in public, people comment on her toned arms. She is proud of her body and she looks fantastic.

Another great aspect of strength training is the fact that you can tailor workouts to achieve the look you want. Even though genetics play a part in how we are shaped (I have my mother's hips), building lean muscle actually changes your body composition, so you can control what gets bigger and what stays smaller. For instance, women with toned, curvy shoulders have intentionally built that muscle.

51

Likewise, women with long, lean muscles have purposely done what was necessary to achieve that look. I already had muscular legs when I started strength training, so I focused on building my shoulders, arms and upper body to appear more symmetrical. If you saw me today, you would not think I had big, bulky "man arms," but curvy, toned arms. This brings us back to the bottom line – women do not get big or manly when they lift weights, unless it is intentional.

The Basics

To start a strength training plan, you need to know the basics. First, it is important to train every major muscle in the body: this includes your chest and back muscles, legs, shoulders, biceps, triceps and abdominals. Even if you need to focus on a specific area more so than others, you still must train every group of muscles. *Lean muscle needs to be completely added in every area of the body.* As mentioned earlier, I have been blessed with muscular legs, but I still have to train them every time I exercise. I just do different exercises with my legs than my arms so one increases in size and the other remains the same size. Again, we are talking about curvature of the muscles, not expansion; your muscles will not expand, they will tone up.

Second, I recommend splitting up your routine so you can focus on different muscle groups throughout the week. Breaking up your strength training plan will allow worked muscles to rest, while reducing the amount of time you spend exercising. When I train clients, we do one day of chest and back exercises and the other day conditioning the shoulder, bicep and triceps muscles. I do, however, target the leg and abdominal muscles on both days. This keeps the workout fun, fresh and exciting.

Third, a focus should always be to increase the stabilizing muscles in the body, which are found in the core muscles. Your core muscles consist of the abdominal, oblique and lower back muscles, and it is an essential part to getting the most out of your strength training routine. Most women begin an exercise program with a trainer, in an exercise class, or by watching a DVD without learning the importance of having a strong, stable core. It is a mistake to participate in any exercise program without first focusing on your core. Having weak core muscles can increase the risk of injury. A strong, stable core will give you better posture and a smaller waistline. You will see your strength increase as you are able to power through more exercises with your rock-hard core. And just so you know, a strong core does not come from doing sit-ups or crunches (thank goodness).

Lastly, you need to do each strength training exercise almost to the point of overwhelm or extreme difficulty. The last two repetitions of each move should be a real challenge. In case you are not familiar with exercise lingo, a "repetition" means one complete movement. Every time you do a bicep curl or a squat, you have just done one repetition. Another term you'll see me use is "set." A "set" is a series of repetitions. So, if you perform 15 bicep curls (or, 15 repetitions), take a break then do another 15 repetitions, you are completing 2 sets of the exercise. With every exercise you do, you should be performing anywhere from 15 to 20 repetitions, doing a total of 2 to 3 sets.

This brings me to another point. New clients ask me, "How

much weight should I use for certain exercises?" My answer is that *weight is relative*. Meaning that the weight I may use for a particular exercise could be different than the weight you need to use. Furthermore, weight used in strength training should be consistently increased. The best way to figure out how much weight you should use is to be sure that the last two repetitions, when completing 15 to 20 repetitions, are very challenging. If you are using 5 pound dumbbells for a bicep curl, attempting to complete 15 repetitions, rep number 14 and 15 should be extremely difficult to manage. If those last two are easy, bump up your dumbbell weight to 8 pounds, and so on.

Let's Sum It Up:

- Lean muscle will make you look small, burn more calories at rest, and feel strong and confident.
- Strength training using body weight, free weights, and exercise or cable machines will not make you big, bulky or masculine. Women who look this way do so intentionally.
- Lean muscle can help to counteract osteoporosis.
- Be sure to strength train *every* muscle in the body each week.
- Do exercises that promote a strong, stable core.
- Perform each exercise close to overwhelm or extreme difficulty. The last two repetitions should be a challenge.

Chapter 9

Using Nutrition to Tackle PCOS

Congratulations on creating an exercise plan and committing to moving your body in a positive way! Pat yourself on the back for doing something that is healthy and beneficial for your body. Exercise may not be easy in the beginning, but it pays off in the end. Now it's time to move on to the next step.

Nutrition is the second step in the "Triple Threat" approach to combating PCOS and insulin resistance. I believe it is the most difficult step to master, but it becomes easier when you take it slow and allow time to create healthy habits. Eating the right foods that promise immunity, balanced hormones and restored health is a lifelong habit, and one that takes some time to figure out based on your lifestyle, habits, and preferences. I will share my knowledge of nutrition, what has worked for me personally, and what other health experts are saying.

I have been learning about nutrition since 2002, and I have never stopped finding, listening or reading the latest information available. I also experiment with everything I recommend for nutrition. These guidelines have been or still are applied in my life and have worked well for me. My main focus for food is to find which combinations produce amazing health benefits. I do not believe in eating to lose weight. I believe our focus should be on long-term health. If your body is balanced and healthy, then excess weight will not be an issue for long. When your body becomes really healthy from the inside-out, body fat will naturally come off. Hear me out on this section, and we'll tie everything together so you can apply it to your personal life.

You are What You Eat

There is so much truth to the saying, "you are what you eat." If you eat fatty foods, you will inevitably become fat. Even if you eat within your "calorie limit," your body will look like the foods you feed it. If you eat squishy doughnuts, you will become soft and squishy, even if you're not heavy. I have some friends, and you probably do, too, who can eat whatever they want and not gain weight. I always feel sorry for these people because they never learn how to eat for long-term health. Being skinny does not mean you are healthy. In fact, you may find that these friends are chronically tired, sick and in general poor health. That's because they eat foods that contribute to poor health. When you follow the motto, "you are what you eat," you will start to view food in a different way. You will choose to eat foods that will give you the most energy, immunity and metabolic boost. Once you are eating this "preventative" diet and eating for health, rather than weight loss, you will feel in control of your body and radiate a glowing confidence. I know because I have women all the time who ask my clients and me what we are doing differently. When you are in control of your health and you feel confident, you will carry yourself differently and people will notice!

Eating for health means you will be choosing foods and eating them in a combination that gives you better digestion. When your bowels are functioning optimally, you flush harmful toxins from the body.

When your digestive system works as it should, you will experience:

✓   clearer skin on your face and body

✓   less bloating .

✓   more energy and stamina

✓   fewer symptoms of PMS

✓   decreased food cravings

✓   better sleep

Stop counting calories

I get that, scientifically speaking, calories matter. If you consume more calories than you burn, you will gain weight. If you burn off more calories than you consume, you will lose weight. This is true, but it is often blown out of proportion.

I took a nutrition class in college and we studied our basal metabolic rate, which is the rate at which your body uses energy (calories) to function, as well as the amount of calories we use doing different daily activities. We also had to do a three day food log to see how many calories we were consuming. I learned that I can consume over 2,100 calories every day and not gain weight; I was not exercising enough for this to be true, but luckily I had done specific things to raise my basal metabolic rate. Burning calories always includes the ones you are burning without exercising. If you are going to focus on the caloric value of anything, concentrate on raising your basal metabolic rate from strength training and eating foods that raise your caloric burn (like protein).

If you focus only on the calories in the foods you eat and not the quality or portion size, you will never, ever keep the weight off. Besides, unless you have the time to keep track of calories consumed, counting calories is boring and complicated. When you eat whole foods, you don't have to count calories, because you are giving your body what it wants and desperately needs. Calories aside, there are foods, like packaged, processed items, that cause health problems and create a mess within your body. It's best to eat foods that will give you vitality, immunity and amazing health so you're naturally losing weight and feeling incredible in your skin.

Let's Sum It Up:
- What you are eating all the time inevitably shows up on the outside.
- Eating for health, both in the short-term and long-term, is the only way to stop obsessing about your weight and heal your body.
- Counting calories is a waste of time; not all calories are created equally.

Chapter 10

You Can Change Your Body Composition

Tosca Reno, author of the *Eat Clean Diet* series, goes by the 80:10:10 rule, stating that a beautiful body is built by 80% of eating the right foods at the right time, 10% by exercising the right way and 10% genetics.[11] I also use this theory when I have clients tell me that they "have always been heavy," or that their "parents were heavy." Just because you may have a family history of disease or obesity does not mean that you're destined to be this way. Exercise and proper nutrition can naturally raise your basal metabolic rate, so you are doing less and burning more without counting calories.

Why not diet?

I do not recommend dieting ever. I consider "dieting" unrealistic because you are not eating the way you will eat for the rest of your life. If you are eating limited, specific foods just so you can temporarily lose weight, you will be in for a nasty surprise when you quit dieting. The weight comes back and, often times, you gain back additional weight!

Put it this way; if you lose 10 pounds in a week or 40 pounds in a month on a strict diet and rigorous exercise program, a large percentage of the weight you lose is made up of water. Most of the water you lose will come back when you start eating the foods you've restricted. Losing too much water weight can also result in dehydration, causing your body to halt any weight loss. Lean muscle is the next thing to go when you lose weight too quickly. Here's why: When your body is starved of the foods (carbohydrates, for one) or calories it needs for energy, it uses up lean muscle. It needs to get the calories from somewhere and lean muscle is the next best thing for it to utilize. In case I wasn't clear in the last chapter, lean muscle helps you burn more calories on a regular basis. Why would you want to lose it? Only a very small percentage of weight loss on rigorous diet and exercise programs is made up of body fat.

Another reason you women gain back all the weight they originally had plus more is because deprivation makes the body go into "starvation mode." When your body senses starvation or deprivation, it believes something is wrong. In response, it works hard to achieve your original weight and sometimes adds a few pounds for safety. Lastly, when you are super deprived on a diet, some women find themselves binging on food they had denied which inevitably adds weight.

Most doctors recommend that you only lose about 2 pounds a week when participating in a weight loss program. I agree. In fact, the longer you take to lose the weight, the longer you will usually keep it off. After slowly losing 5 pounds, your body becomes used to the "new you," and it makes appropriate changes to maintain your new weight.

Usually losing weight the right way takes a little longer. But, is 6 to 12 months really that long? Making lifestyle changes the right way takes time, but it's long-lasting. Please don't be fooled by partaking in an impractical and ineffective "diet program."

Diets are too strict.

Dieting doesn't work for a few reasons: diets are too strict, too complicated, and most often do not keep your health in mind. In my nutrition class in college I was in a debate group that argued the pros of a certain "no to carbs – yes to bacon" diet, and we won. I focused on all the good things about the diet, like how it includes vegetables and instructs the dieter to refrain from starchy and refined carbohydrates. Our argument was convincing, but what we did not mention was the fact that a high percentage of this particular diet's participants gained all of the lost weight back, plus more, once they started eating carbohydrates again. The main reason was that most people cannot permanently cut carbohydrates from their diet. On occasion I have a client who is ready to do anything to lose weight and decides to cut out a certain food group. I respond by asking if they will be able to cut that food group out for the rest of their lives. If they cannot cut it out for life, they will regain weight once they begin eating the particular food again.

There are special instances when it's perfectly alright to cut out certain foods from your diet. I am lactose intolerant, and I have not eaten cheese since 2007. I also do not think dairy products are good for us (side note: I do not eat most milk products 90% of the time). The point is that if you can do it for life, go ahead. If you cannot, find a way to minimize it from your diet. Also, be sure you aren't cutting out a healthy group of foods like carbohydrate. As you will learn in the next chapter, some carbohydrates, like whole grains, vegetables and fruits, are healthy and beneficial to you.

Diets are too complicated.

Diets are too complicated to incorporate into everyday life. Your diet must be easy to adhere to anywhere you go. If you are on a cruise or at a friend's home, you must be able to live and eat the same diet all the time. Can you do this with a low-carb / no-carb diet? If you can, kudos to you. I cannot follow any one diet. And even if I could, I would feel deprived. The key is live out a plan that is easy to understand without obsessing about what you're eating or what the scale reads.

Diets do not keep your long-term health in mind.

An eating plan should have your health in mind. I have one friend who insists on a particular diet recommended by an online fitness trainer who has you cut out carbs (including fruit) and drink diet soda. I was not surprised to find out that she was in poor health from cutting out healthy carbs. She also had trouble staying on the diet and therefore gained all of the excess weight back, after she stopped participating in the diet. Her metabolism was completely screwed up, and she couldn't figure out why. I will tell you the same thing I told her, "Do not follow a diet plan that does not have your long-term health in mind!" In all of the research I have done, I have never found that cutting out essential carbs and drinking diet soda will help create amazing health benefits. If you're unhealthy on the inside, it will eventually show on the outside.

Diets that are quick-fixes, making you cut out healthy food groups, instilling complicated rules, and not keeping your long-term health in mind are a recipe for disaster. If you are ever tempted by one of these diets, just keep in mind that if you cannot do it for life you will be in a worse off once you stop it. You will likely gain more weight once stopping the diet program, and you may find that your metabolism does not function properly.

If you are currently on a diet or just got off one, read on and learn how you can naturally and easily restore your metabolism and undo any damage on your body.

Let's Sum It Up:

- The way you look is 80% what you're eating, 10% efforts from exercise and 10% genetics. This is great news when you're eating right!
- Never go on an unrealistic "diet" that cuts out healthy food groups.
- Most diets cause the dieter to gain all of the weight back plus more after going off the diet.
- Diets usually do not work because they are too complicated, too strict and do not keep your long-term health in mind.
- Strict diets can screw up your metabolism and hormones, making it

You *Can* Change Your Body Composition

a real challenge to lose weight in the future.

Chapter 11

Eating Right is E.A.S.Y.

Eating right is not as complicated as every "diet" book has made it seem. Eating right seems difficult at first, but only because it is a new idea and it takes time to become part of your life.

Have you ever wanted something so badly, knowing it would take some work and effort on your part, but the pay off would be worth it? That's what eating right is like. Learning these nutrition principles are foreign to some women in the beginning, but with a little effort and consistency, the rewards are great. The end result makes the effort you put in worth it.

I remember joining a Toastmasters Club a few years ago. My husband wanted to improve his public speaking skills and suggested I join with him. I remember dreading the thought of speaking in front of a group of at least 30 people every week. Even if I did not give a speech, I would likely be called on at the end of each meeting for "Table Topics," where members are randomly selected to come to the front of the room and respond to the speaker's question or statement. During "Table Topics," the speaker could be touching on a topic such as politics, and after doing an introduction to their topic, they would say, "Katie, how do you feel about the President's stand on [fill in the blank]?" Can you imagine being called on and having to give an impromptu speech for at least 60 seconds, in front of 30 strangers?

Eating Right is E.A.S.Y.

As scary and complex as constructing speeches and mastering the "put on the spot" nervous feeling seemed, this was something that would make me a better speaker and conversationalist. So I joined.

I was called up for Table Topics at my first meeting, and I think I stood up there for 20 seconds before turning bright red and bee-lining for my seat. After that experience, I took the necessary time to make Toastmasters a part of my life. As you can see, I was a novice in the beginning. Speaking in front of others was something that I had little experience with and did not do effectively. So I put in the work, time and energy to overcome my fear and frustration, and it was worth it in the end. Within 2 months, I won the "Best Table Topics, Best Speaker and Best Evaluator" awards. I now love to speak in public and sincerely believe it positively impacts others around me.

So many women become lazy and complacent about eating right because it takes work, time and energy, and it doesn't seem worth it to them. So, they go on a strict diet, compromising their health and inevitably failing and feeling ashamed, embarrassed and frustrated – just as I did when I bombed during my first Table Topics. These women are wasting precious time by participating in a strict diet when they could be using that time to learn a new way of eating. It is so easy once you give it time and dedicate yourself to learning and applying my strategies.

Will you mess up and eat badly? For sure. Just as I messed up on my first speech in Toastmasters (I turned red and cried afterwards), you will inevitably eat something that is not good for you. Screwing up is part of the process, and it is good for you. When you mess up and eat something that doesn't align with what I teach you, you will learn from it and remember why you don't want to eat it anymore.

Screwing up in Toastmasters pushed me to do it the right way, by following the rules to construct and memorize good speeches. Once I mastered it, I could do things more efficiently, in less time, and get better results. This is the same principle with eating right – making mistakes will help you learn tweak you're eating so you're getting better results in less time. When referring to his many failed attempts at inventing the light bulb, Thomas Edison commented, "I did not fail 1000 times. I successfully found 1000 ways that the light bulb would not work."

I still occasionally eat foods that are not part of the program I teach, but I learn from it and move on. As an example, my husband and I bought brownie mix and icing ingredients a while back. Yes, all of the ingredients were organic, but it still contained sugar in some form. I also had about five brownies! The point is that I won't be eating those again for a really long time. I didn't feel sick or like I gained weight, but there is a reason I try not to overdo it on sugar and now I know why: I want my body to be a strong, healthy, energetic temple. The point is that it is okay to make mistakes. You don't have to be perfect. Eating perfectly is not always plausible, nor is it necessary for losing weight with PCOS.

Will it be difficult? Some parts will be difficult to apply and others will be simple. The important thing to remember is consistency. I was not a good speaker overnight; it took several months to be comfortable in front of others. When I won "Best Speaker" for a recycling speech that was 5 minutes long, I practiced the speech at least 20 times over a 2 week period. I did a great job on my speech because I worked my tush off for it! You have your whole life to improve and tweak your diet to make it fit for you, your family and your lifestyle. I did not start eating right overnight. It took time for me to slowly incorporate healthy habits into my everyday life. Once a habit would become "second nature" and a part of my lifestyle, I would master another.

Eating right can become a part of your lifestyle. Just remember to make it a priority! To easily remember how to eat from now on, just remember to eat the E.A.S.Y. way. Eat every three to four hours; Always combine a protein and carbohydrate; Stay away from harmful foods; and You're allowed to have treats. We will discuss these in depth in the upcoming chapters. Stay tuned!

Let's Sum It Up:
- Eating right takes time to become a part of your lifestyle.
- The most important aspect of good nutrition is consistency. No matter how much you mess up, sticking with your plan is the key.
- Eat the E.A.S.Y. way for best results.
- Eat every three to four hours.
- Always combine a protein and carbohydrate.
- Stay away from harmful foods.
- You're allowed to have treats.

Chapter 12

Eat Every Three to Four Hours

Eating every few hours creates steady blood sugar levels and increases your basal metabolic rate. Remember earlier when I wrote about your basal metabolic rate (BMR) and how it is the best way to burn maximum calories so you don't have to exercise as much? Eating often ensures your body is using up energy to digest and process the 4 or 5 meals you eat throughout the day, thus your BMR increases.[11]

Your body is a very smart machine that was designed to withstand times of famine by storing fat to conserve energy. If you go longer than 4 hours without refueling your body with proper nutrition, it will in turn store body fat to protect you. Think about it the "caveman days"; we weren't originally created to withstand the stressful, fast-paced environment of modern technology. *After going longer than 4 hours without eating, your body is under the impression that if you are not eating it is because there is no food.* To ensure your safety, your body shuts down and goes into fat-storing mode so that you can survive. There are intricate systems within the body that need to function in order for your survival. Your body does not care that you want to lose weight for your vacation. If you are not giving it the fuel it needs to keep your heart ticking and organs properly running, it will store fat to get the job done. That is why we can physically go without food for 40 days. Your body knows how to survive in the case that food cannot be found. When you feed your body throughout the day, you are indicating that you will continue to give it the fuel it needs to function. In return, your metabolism will increase and your body will start burning fat as calories are being used.

Eating often guarantees blood sugar levels are steady and will not spike drastically then drop. This also means that food cravings are kept to a minimum. Michael Lewis, a writer for Men's Health, notes in *Control Your Cravings*, "cravings are all about blood sugar. If your levels are consistent throughout the day your eating patterns will be also. But when you starve yourself for hours, cravings start calling. And trust me, you will answer." Craving sugar, refined carbs and alcohol is the biggest enemy to weight loss. The sooner you can get your cravings under control, the quicker you can be in control of your weight.[12]

Frequent eating also means you will have constant, clean energy. No more mid-afternoon energy dips from starvation or heavy, carb-laden lunches. You will be able to think more clearly, stay more focused and accomplish more.

In addition, consistent energy will improve your moods. Have you ever witnessed a friend who starved herself to lose weight and was impossible to be around? Crankiness and irritability can come from not eating enough food. When you fuel your body 4 to 6 times a day, you will be in control of your moods and attitude.[11]

The best side effect of eating 4 to 5 meals a day is that your body composition will change dramatically. *You will look more toned and feel slimmer.* When I started to consistently eat every 3 hours, I was able to see results from my strength training efforts within 2 weeks! I could notice more definition in my abs, arms and butt.

Start by eating breakfast within an hour of waking up. Breakfast fuels you for the day and there is more than enough evidence that eating breakfast is associated with weight loss. Studies show that men and women who eat breakfast are less likely to overeat at the end of the day.

Eating breakfast is closely associated with weight management. A report from WebMD entitled, "Lose Weight: Eat Breakfast," claims that people who have lost 30 pounds or more and kept it off for at least a year (some as long as six years), all had the common habit of eating breakfast every day.[13]

If the thought of eating a meal first thing in the morning nauseates you, try eating something small like a smoothie or a piece of toast with some almond butter. Just be sure to eat a combination of protein and carbohydrates and make it healthy.

Let's Sum It Up:
- Eating every 3 to 4 hours increases basal metabolic rate and burns more calories throughout the day.
- Withholding food from the body after 4 hours can lead to fat storage.
- Eating every few hours reduces cravings for unhealthy foods.
- Eating often increases energy, focus and mental clarity and improves moods.
- Start the day by eating breakfast. This will promote weight loss.

71

Chapter 13

Always Combine Protein and Carbohydrates

Eating a protein and carbohydrate together ensures you are burning fat and retaining any lean muscle from strength training. Eating in this fashion also helps reduce cravings. When you combine your foods like this, you will feel less hungry and more in control of your food choices.[11]

Protein

Protein is good for metabolic function as it increases your ability to burn calories. It is the necessary building block to gain lean muscle as a result of strength training. As discussed earlier, the more lean muscle you retain, the longer, leaner, and stronger you will be.

It is also beneficial for the nervous and immune system to function properly. Protein is necessary to develop antibodies that improve the ability to ward off any illness. Consuming protein contributes to hair and nail growth (who doesn't want that?), and it aids in the recovery of wounds and scars. Protein is also the macronutrient that keeps you full and satisfied after a meal.

Always Combine Protein and Carbohydrates

Protein can include meat, fish, seafood, eggs, beans, legumes, nuts, dairy, and tofu. You can eat a vegetarian or an animal protein at every meal – just be vigilant of portion sizes. If you are eating red meat, poultry or fish, eat about 3 to 5 ounces or the size of the palm of your hand. When eating eggs, I usually eat 1 egg and 2 to 3 egg whites. Beans and legumes should be eaten in ½ cup servings; these can also count as a carbohydrate. Nuts and seeds should all be eaten in moderation. Eat about 2 to 3 ounces of nuts at any given meal. Although I do not recommend eating large amounts of dairy (re: cheese), 8 ounces is an appropriate serving size for milk. Tofu and Tempeh can be eaten in various amounts, and you can find the serving size amount on the package. This serving size will vary based on how much protein you want to consume.

We women should not be eating more than 30 grams of protein at any given meal. Consuming 30 grams is *a lot* of protein. If you consume more 30 grams of protein at one meal, the body will usually store it as fat. I recommend eating about 10 to 20 grams of protein at each meal. This is really easy to achieve, based on portion sizes. This book's Appendix provides a protein chart, naming healthy protein choices as well as appropriate portion sizes.

Let's Sum It Up:
- Eating a combo of protein and carbohydrates at every meal increases the body's fat-burning ability and reduces cravings for junk foods.
- Protein has many health benefits including increased metabolism,

increased immunity and it keeps you satisfied after a meal.

- Protein aids in the growth of healthy hair and nails, and recovery of wounds and scars.

- Protein choices can include meat, fish, eggs, beans, legumes, nuts, dairy and tofu.

- Eat the appropriate serving size for protein, getting no more than 30 grams at each meal.

Carbohydrates

Carbohydrates provide our main source of energy. I know there are diets on the market that tell you to cut out carbs. Try it and you will see that in a short time you become cranky, irritable and downright witchy! Studies show that consuming carbohydrates keeps the brain chemical, serotonin, functioning at an optimal level. Serotonin is responsible for positively affecting your mood, thoughts and behavior by promoting feelings of joy, optimism and relaxation.[14] *Conversely, when we restrict or refuse carbohydrates from our diet, we can become depressed, irritable and more likely to overeat and indulge our cravings.*

Carbs provide the brainpower we need to concentrate, think clearly, and control mood swings. We need them to maintain our mental sanity and stay in a good mood.

Insoluble and soluble fiber is needed to gain the many benefits of eating carbohydrates. They also contribute to weight loss and support a healthy digestive system. Fiber found in carbs is either indigestible or digested slowly. Both types of fiber cause blood glucose and insulin to remain at a steady level, allowing the body to burn sugar instead of storing it as fat.[14]

You see, most women with PCOS find it easy to gain weight and challenging to lose it because of insulin resistance. Most likely, the cells in your body are resistant to the insulin and glucose being produced, so both are free floating in the body. This not only causes further hormonal imbalance, but it makes it difficult to control cravings, lose weight and burn body fat.

You must learn to retrain the body to use carbohydrates as energy without storing it as fat. Most likely, you are experiencing the latter situation and almost everything you eat is being stored as body fat. Eating certain carbohydrates in small portions at specific times will help counteract this problem. This will allow your body to begin functioning as a fat-burning machine. When you eat the nutritious, healthy version of your favorite carbs, you will reduce any cravings for the unhealthy ones.

Carbohydrates are broken down into 3 simple categories: 1) grains, 2) vegetables and 3) fruit.

Grains can include oats, brown rice, and any type of whole grains like amaranth, quinoa (pronounced "keen-wah") and whole wheat. Choosing produce is easy because I recommend eating all vegetables and fruit. I do not, nor will I ever, recommend cutting out any fruit or vegetable; they all have essential vitamins, minerals and nutrients, and they are a part of a healthy diet.

Serving sizes are important with grains and starchy vegetables because of the insulin required to digest these foods. I recommend eating a ½ cup of whole grains like brown rice, whole grain pasta or oatmeal, 1 slice of whole grain bread, English muffin or bagel, and 4 ounces of starchy vegetables like potatoes.

Appropriate portions for vegetables and fruits can be found in the Glycemic Index. The Glycemic Index (GI) determines the effect a carbohydrate has on your blood sugar and insulin levels (the website to the GI list is in the Appendix). The lower the number on the chart, the better the effect it has on your body as it takes longer to break down and requires less insulin production. The foods that have a lower number are considered low-glycemic. If the food is higher on the GI, however, your blood sugar spikes as it tries too quickly to break down the food, thus your pancreas secretes high amounts of insulin.[14]

Foods that are lower on the GI can be eaten in higher quantities. Overeating on broccoli will not make you gain weight, nor will it have a negative impact on your health. Foods that are higher on the GI should be eaten in moderation; watermelon is good for you, but shouldn't be eaten every day in large quantities.[15]

Let's Sum It Up:
- Carbohydrates contribute to weight loss, optimal digestion and the brainpower we need to concentrate and control moods.
- Carbohydrates include whole grains, vegetables and fruits.
- Appropriate serving sizes depends on how the carbohydrate is rated on the Glycemic Index, which determines the effect a carb has on blood sugar and insulin levels.

Chapter 14

Fats and Organics: Why The
Make You Thin

Good fats are highly nutritious but are not mentioned as much b(
I don't want to bombard you with too much information (too
right?). Good fats are a macronutrient that can be added to 1
throughout the day. They don't need to be included in every meal
protein and carbohydrates. I have read many books that tell yo
combine all three (protein, carbohydrates and fat) to each of your r
meals, but I think it's too much information to keep in mi
Personally, I always eat a protein and carbohydrate, and I sprin
good fats in some of those meals.

There are many reasons why you should be eating good fat
Eating good fats can help prevent heart disease and blockage caused b
high cholesterol. It is crazy to think that most of us don't know tha
"fat" as a food can either be healthy and helpful when shedding bod'
fat or it can be detrimental and deadly to our health. This comes dowi
to which types of "fat" you are eating.

According to the American Heart Association (AHA), eating
healthy, mono- or poly-unsaturated fats can help reduce ba(
cholesterol and "help your body get rid of newly formed cholesterol.'
In case you are unaware, high cholesterol is a major factor in coronary

heart disease and can lead to a heart attack. If you remember in an earlier chapter, women with PCOS are *4* to *7* times more likely to have a heart attack, and we are prone to high blood pressure and high cholesterol!

These are the fats the AHA recommends you use: olive oil, other nut and seed oils (like walnut, almond and sesame seed oil), nuts, seeds, and avocados. Eating these fats in moderation can also help you burn off the other type of fat (re: body fat and cellulite).

Good fats like olive, walnut, almond, and sesame oils, nuts, seeds, and avocados should be eaten at various meals throughout the week. It's best to consume them in smaller portions and at their original temperature (don't fry food with oil). Healthy serving sizes include 1 to 2 tablespoons for oil, a handful for nuts and seeds (or 2 to 3 ounces), and ½ avocado.

Let's Sum It Up:
- Good fats should be eaten in various meals throughout the week.
- Good fats can reduce cholesterol and may prevent the risk of a heart attack.
- These fats help shed unwanted body fat and cellulite.
- Eat good fats in smaller portions.

Eat Organic

I do have one particular principle that I rarely ignore: eat organic animal products. We women with PCOS cannot afford to deal with any further complications in our hormonal health. Non-organic animal products are chock full of unnatural, harmful antibiotics and hormones. I am referring to meat, including chicken and red meat, as well as dairy products. Believe me; it will cost you far less in the long-term to pay for organic meat and dairy products now.

In his bestselling book, *Natural Cures "They" Don't Want You to Know About*, Kevin Trudeau explains the difference between organic and non-organic animal products. Organic animals, while they are alive, have genetics that are in their most natural state, are not given any type of drugs, and are allowed to consume naturally while roaming freely. *Non-organic animals, on the other hand, have been genetically modified in breeding.* They are injected with growth hormones and antibiotics, are not allowed to roam freely, fed an unnatural diet of chemicals as well as ground up parts of other animals.[9] I won't go into any further detail because this subject completely makes me sick. I have read one too many times the inhumane, disgusting, despicable practices performed in non-organic farms.

If you're eating non-organic meat, you are consuming everything that was given to the animal, including the antibiotics, hormones and additives in the animal's food. This is why I believe we should strive to eat only the most organic, natural meat available. If you want more horrifying information about eating non-organic animals, I suggest you read Rory Freedman and Kim Barnouin's book, *Skinny Bitch*.

As you may guess, I also suggest you purchase organic produce. Dr. Don Colbert notes in *Toxic Relief* that pesticides found in non-organic produce have been linked to higher amounts of xenoestrogen in women. Xenoestrogen acts as a "counterfeit" of estrogen, causing hormonal imbalance and leading to serious conditions—such as fibrocystic breast diseases and endometriosis. These synthetic hormones may even contribute to breast cancer and endometrial cancer.[17]

Dr. Colbert also notes that fruits and vegetables are not the only place we can easily consume deadly pesticides. He says, "When we bite into a fatty piece of steak, a greasy hamburger, sausages, bacon or even butter and cream, we are ingesting even more pesticide residues." These pesticides are being stored in our body, mostly in our "fatty tissue." They create an unhealthy environment and cause the body to develop sickness, disease and possibly long-term illness.[17]

According to the U.S. Department of Health and Human Services, PCOS may cause endometrial cancer as a result of a lack of progesterone being produced in the body. This government website states, "Without progesterone, the endometrium becomes thick, which can cause heavy bleeding or irregular bleeding. Over time, this can lead to endometrial hyperplasia when the lining grows too much, and cancer."

Choosing to pay a little extra for organic foods will give you the safe, healthy nutrients your body needs to rebalance. Think of it as an investment in your health. Whenever my older brother complains about spending extra on organic food, I remind him that a long-term health problem will cost him far more. For the sake of your physical and emotional health, spend the money on organic foods.

If you cannot afford organic foods, cut back on certain grocery items, and spring for organic meat and dairy products. I would even recommend buying the meat that is nonorganic if it states that it is free from hormonal and antibiotic injections. These products aren't as good as organic ones, but they are better than consuming synthetic chemicals and hormones. There are also affordable choices at large warehouse stores like Costco in which you can find frozen, organic meat and wild caught fish.

If you have the extra cash, start by buying the organic fruits and vegetables with an edible peel. For instance, apples, pears, and spinach all are without a thick, outer layer and therefore more likely to absorb pesticides. Organic oranges, bananas and grapefruits can always be purchased when you have a bigger budget. When having to choose, it's best to purchase these foods with an "edible peel" (like apples, pears and spinach) first. You can also research local co-ops that allow you to purchase organic food in bulk with a group, saving you cash on healthy groceries. There is also the option of growing your own vegetables or visiting local farmers' markets to purchase affordable organic produce.

If you do not have access to organic foods, there are many online grocers and suppliers that will ship organic foods to your door. They are more expensive, but worth it if you have the budget.

Let's Sum It Up:
- Organic foods are essential to rebalance and restore hormonal health.

- Nonorganic animals are often treated inhumanely, are injected with growth hormones and antibiotics to make them grow bigger and fatter faster.

- Nonorganic produce has been shown to be full of harmful pesticides that contribute to poor health and possible disease and illness.

- Women with PCOS are already susceptible to the diseases and conditions to which nonorganic foods may contribute.

- If you do not have money for organic, cut back on some groceries and only buy organic meat and dairy products.

- When purchasing organic produce, to save on cash, buy only the fruits and vegetables that have an "edible peel" like apples, pears and spinach.

- You can become a part of a local co-op to purchase organic foods in bulk and save money.

- Local farmers' markets have affordable organic produce.

Chapter 15

Stay Away from Harmful Foods

Eating a protein and carbohydrate every 3 to 4 hours will give you tremendous health benefits and will also keep you from eating junk foods. There are certain foods that contribute to poor health, and we want to do whatever it takes to eat as little of these foods as possible. Combining nutraceuticals in Step 3 (we'll get to that later) will help you control your cravings and hunger for nasty, disease-causing garbage food. Plus, the less you eat of these foods, the less you will crave them.

Most harmful foods come in the form of a package. Packaged foods automatically indicate that there is something unnatural about it. Think in terms of cereals, candy, soda and lunch meat. Unless the food is in its original form like meat, eggs, whole grains, vegetables or fruit, chances are it has been processed.

The reason most processed foods are bad for our bodies lies in the description. A "processed" food is just that: it was altered from its original, natural, healthy state and turned into something that could taste better and last longer. Think about how our bodies were created. We were designed to be able to eat the foods on this earth. We were given the vegetables, grains, fruit and meat required to sustain our health. Over time, companies focused on turning larger profits have chemically altered their food, making it tastier to eat, easier to make, and easier to sell on a large scale. These foods are what have made our culture fat, unhealthy and plagued with health problems.

That's the big, dirty secret of the food industry – that these additives and unnatural substances used in foods are making our world so darn unhealthy.[9]

I do not spend a lot of time teaching about the foods you shouldn't be eating because I think it focuses on the negative. Whatever you focus on, you get more of. In a nutshell, foods that are not good for you, ones that cause serious health problems, are usually made by "man" and chemically altered in some way to look, taste and smell better. This is so we become addicted to these foods. You already know what they are, but just for kicks, I will list them anyway.[16]

Stay away from these foods as much as possible:
- Fried foods
- Cheese
- Pastries, doughnuts, cookies, candy, cakes and pies
- Pork (if it's organic, you make the choice, but I consider pork an "unclean" animal because of the foods the pig is given and the environment in which it thrives)

Stay away from these ingredients as much as possible:
- High fructose corn syrup
- Hydrogenated or partially hydrogenated oils
- Food dyes and colorings, such as Red 40

- Additives and preservatives (these are even found in lunch meat!)
- Fake sugar and aspartame (this includes Splenda)
- Bleached or "enriched" flour

All of the above foods and ingredients have damaging effects on the body. If you want more evidence that they are disease-causing, insulin-spiking, fattening foods, I, again, suggest that you read the book, *Skinny Bitch*, or Kevin Trudeau's, *Natural Weight Loss Cures "They" Don't Want You to Know About*. I'm always going to ask that you treat your body well by giving it what it wants most: whole, natural foods. Anything that the body does not "recognize" (re: I didn't say "digest"), is either stored as fat or flushed, leaving traces of chemicals, toxins and harmful substances.

Again, I don't like to focus too much on what we shouldn't be eating. If you are eating enough of the right foods all the time, you won't be hungry for or crave the unhealthy stuff. If you're feeling upset or angry (be honest) at the fact that I may have named some of your favorite foods as unhealthy and something you should think of giving up, read on. I know the next chapter will make you happy.

Start Reading Labels

The best way to get started making better food choices is to read labels and choose "whole" foods. Labels will tell you everything you need to know about packaged foods. Most people read the content containing the amount of calories or sugar a specific food contains. I go straight to the ingredients. If something contains only 20 calories per serving, but the first ingredient is high fructose corn syrup, forget it! There is no way I will put that in my body. If you want to learn how to read labels, just look at the ingredient list. If you can't pronounce an ingredient or if it sounds unnatural, skip it. A good example would be to look at a typical "protein bar" – there are about 30 ingredients, and most of those ingredients are unrecognizable. Most of the choices for protein bars are garbage. Skip them. Usually packaged foods at natural food stores have cleaner and healthier ingredients.

By the way, if you're unsure what "whole" means, just remember personal trainer Jillian Michael's saying: "If it came from the ground or it had a mother, it's whole."[8] Gross, but easy to remember.

When making healthy choices in your diet, small changes add up to big results. When you do make small, but consistent choices, you may barely notice your eating habits are changing for the better. Approach your significant other, family and friends and ask them to be supportive of the changes you are trying to make. Remember, this is your body and you are the one who has to fight for it. No one else can do it for you. Stay strong and persevere when everyone else is eating whatever they want all the time. Look at that person and decide if you want to be like them. Think about their decision to eat poorly. The pain of changing your diet is far easier to deal with than the pain of living with PCOS and its symptoms. Make the choice and stick with it.

Let's Sum It Up:
- Making small changes in your diet can add up to BIG results.

- Foods that are not whole or natural are not recognized by the body and can cause serious, long-term health consequences.
- Chemically altered foods were originally created this way so that manufacturing companies could spend less money producing larger quantities of addictive foods.
- Focus on foods you should be eating instead of the unhealthy ones.
- Become a label-reading whiz by focusing on ingredients instead of calories.

Chapter 16

You're Allowed to Eat Treats

Yes, you heard me right! As contradictory as it sounds (especially after the last several chapters), treats are part of the "Triple Threat" approach. I love treats. I enjoy them on a Friday night or during the holidays. Treats, in and of themselves, do not make you fat, nor do they contribute to poor health. It is the *type* of treats, and the amount, that do damage to the body.

Here is what defines a treat: any food outside of my good choices for protein, carbohydrates, and good fats. If a large food corporation chemically altered it, it is not whole. Know what I mean? Strawberry Italian ice is not whole. Spinach dip isn't either. If it's not whole, consider it a treat.

Whenever I decide to eat something that isn't so healthy, I simply follow a format that helps ensure these foods do not harm my health or my hard-earned weight loss progress. If you find you would like to eat a treat, be sure to apply the following guidelines.

Do you really want a treat, or are you eating your emotions?

Whenever I want some chocolate, I first decide whether or not my desire is because chocolate would be the most delicious thing to eat at the moment, or if I am angry, hurt, frustrated, sad, or feeling some other emotion that I will bury inside by eating a piece of chocolate. Sometimes just asking myself this question keeps me from eating any chocolate. There have been times when I realized that my stress from an encounter with someone left me wanting to drown my overwhelmed spirit in a huge chocolate pie. Other times I admitted to myself that eating the chocolate would make me feel "fat," and would therefore be my "punishment" for being such a lousy wife, friend or coach. The truth is that many times we think we want treats, but what we *really need* is prayer or a hug.

If you can get into the habit of asking yourself some simple questions before diving into a huge piece of pizza or pie, you will often turn it down. Not to mention, this one exercise will gradually allow you to be more in tune with your body; being mindful of your emotions will help you lose weight in the long run.

If you really want that yummy treat, eat it slowly and enjoy every single bite.

Inhaling your food usually leads to overeating and eventual weight gain. One of the huge culprits of insulin resistance is shoveling food down your throat. Your body was not designed to produce the amount of insulin required to digest massive amounts of food in a short amount of time. Plus, when you decide to indulge in a treat, you should be savoring every morsel.

Life is too short to say no to dessert. So, when I eat a treat, I chew slowly and taste every yummy ingredient. When you eat like this, you are sending a message to your brain that says *I am allowed to eat treats*. When you give yourself the big approval to eat dessert or other treats, they don't seem as taboo and are therefore less appealing.

Don't get me wrong, I love homemade chocolate chip cookies, but because no one, not even me, can tell me that I am not allowed to have one (or five), I usually have two or three and I am satisfied. In the past, when I felt like I could "never eat badly," I would secretly eat about 20 cookies in one sitting. Feel my pain? Start telling yourself and your friends and family that you are allowed to eat treats. My husband initially had a hard time hearing this from me. After all, here I was, a weight loss coach, and I was eating dessert whenever I wanted. The real truth is that he needed to come to a place where he wasn't always judging his own decisions to eat the occasional treat. You see? Feeling guilty about having a treat is an emotion that does not serve you. If you decide that you will never eat dessert again, then so be it. For the rest of the population, we need only eat dessert when we want it, and we need to be eating it slowly enough to enjoy every last bit.

More often than not, opt to eat the healthier version of your treat.

You may have already caught on that I love sweet stuff. It's true. I am such a sucker for anything with sugar. However, I know better than to eat refined sugar and flour all the time. What I learned to do a long time ago was to choose a healthier version of all of my favorite treats. For instance, whenever I make chocolate chip cookies, I buy Bob's Red Mill cookie mix. It contains organic, gluten-free ingredients and is free from dairy, egg and peanut by-products. I also use Earth Balance vegan butter, organic, free-range eggs and almond milk to make them, so they are as healthy as chocolate chip cookies can get. My husband and his brother absolutely love them!

When my husband and I have a "pizza" night, we usually make them with a whole grain or sometimes gluten-free crust and put our own toppings on them. My husband loves pizza, and it sure beats the yucky, greasy pizza pies you get from delivery.

When you start figuring out how to make your favorite treats healthily, you will love how fun it is to still eat the things you love without any guilt! Most of the time, I just cut back on certain ingredients, like butter and cream, to tweak recipes and make them more healthy.

Nix the treats you don't really enjoy for the ones you LOVE.

My husband loves to drink wine at special events and holidays. He considers this his "indulgent treat," and will opt to have wine over dessert if it is a choice. I am the complete opposite. I usually turn down wine if I have to choose between it and the dessert table. I don't waste my time eating both because I won't feel badly about eating a treat when I didn't have the added calories of the wine. Likewise, if I am choosing from someone's dessert table at Thanksgiving, I will only take small amounts of the things I know I want. I don't want to waste my "treat bucket" on things I don't really enjoy. Get it?

Start saying no to the things you don't love so you can have what you really want. Put it this way, if you had a $100 gift certificate to your favorite shoe store, would you spend it on the first two pair of shoes the attendant showed you, or you would you save it for the perfect pair? I know the black flats are the first thing you saw, but wouldn't you rather have the sexy boots? Why spend the money on something you don't really want when you know you'll feel amazing wearing your new boots? Likewise, why waste your time on foods you don't absolutely love? Save it for what you want. This also works when you go out to eat. I always, always say no to the bread basket because, truly, bread does nothing for me. Most people will eat it because it's there; I know better. I save my "treat bucket" for wine or a dessert.

The best way to start implementing this tactic is to practice saying "no." "No thank you, I'm fine/full/not interested." Say it if you don't want it. Gaining weight because you say "yes" to everything is far worse than hurting someone's feeling when you turn down their homemade cupcakes for the twentieth time.

I learned a long time ago that this "eating healthy" idea is a lifelong commitment. If I am going to eat healthily long-term, then I need to enjoy it and benefit from it. Having this kind of outlook in regard to your diet can help you ease up and relax about the choices you make. You do not have to be perfect all the time, but you do have to be aware of what you are eating. Being rigid in your meal choices will set you up for disaster because you will inevitably feel deprived and angry that you cannot have the things you want when you want them. I am very conscious of the foods I put in my body. I eat as many healthy foods as often as possible so that when I want a less-than-healthy treat, it doesn't impact my health or the scale.

Let's Sum It Up:

- Eating treats is encouraged; as part of a lifelong diet plan, treats should be eaten to avoid the feeling of deprivation.
- Decide whether or not you *really* want a treat, or if you are eating to soothe emotions.
- Eat treats slowly and enjoy every single bite.
- Whenever possible, eat a healthier version of your treat to avoid the harmful ingredients mentioned earlier.
- Say "no" to the treats you don't love so you can eat the ones you really want without feeling guilty.

Chapter 17

Nutraceuticals: My Secret Weapon

Congratulations on making it to the third step in the "Triple Threat" approach to overcome PCOS! I'm so proud you are making healthy changes. Now that you are aware of the positive impact regular exercise and healthy foods can have on PCOS and insulin resistance, it's time to learn the final step that will kick PCOS to the curb.

Since being diagnosed with PCOS, have you already tried to exercise and eat healthily and found that it is next to impossible to lose a pound? In fact, maybe you have grown tired of trying to lose weight the "natural way" so you quit exercising and now eat whatever you want, only to find that you gain weight easily. The classic prescription for weight loss that doctors and experts give to people who need to lose weight is: "eat right and exercise." Unfortunately, most women with PCOS cannot apply this principle and be successful. As I mentioned earlier, most women with PCOS also have insulin resistance. This simply means that your body is not properly utilizing the glucose and insulin being produced, so it is free-floating throughout the body. Therefore, only a small amount of exercising and nutritious foods will allow you to lose weight until you address this issue. You must find a way to reverse the effects of insulin resistance. Otherwise, you will find that you cannot lose weight and putting on weight is a cinch. I used to be there, too. Now, I do not gain weight, and I find it very easy to lose weight when I need to.

I was already exercising and eating healthily when I discovered supplements, also called nutraceuticals (vitamins, minerals and herbs that are disease-specific), which address PCOS and insulin resistance. I now consider these supplements to be my "secret ingredient" and I am very passionate about telling other women with PCOS about them. Don't be mistaken, you will not likely see great benefits if you take these supplements and then don't exercise or eat right; these things must be done in accordance, combining all three steps. However, if you make small changes in steps 1 and 2, and incorporate taking supplements, you will see changes.

I find that nutraceuticals and natural supplements allow the body to naturally restore its systems so the root cause of PCOS and insulin resistance is effectively addressed and resolved.

To this day, I only take my supplements occasionally. I don't have to take them every day, nor do I feel my body needs them. When I first discovered nutraceuticals, I decided to take them religiously for a maximum of a few years. Now, my body does what it is supposed to; it provides me with so much immunity, vitality and abundant health. If the supplements you choose are effective, you shouldn't have to take them forever. *Supplements are a means to an end and should be taken to help your body naturally reverse PCOS and insulin resistance.*

Hear me out: we need the right exercises and specific foods, but PCOS and insulin resistance are complicated and cannot always be overcome with just exercise and diet. We need additional help. Since most available foods do not contain a concentrated amount of the nutrients to balance and restore hormones in a body with PCOS, we must look to another source.

The reason I prefer natural supplements is because the ingredients are closest to their original state (as a whole food), so they are recognized and properly utilized by the body (this is only the case when buying from a reputable company or brand). As an example, when consuming Vitamin C, Milk Thistle or Chromium, the body instantly processes these healing vitamins, minerals and herbs. They are whole nutrients that God gave us to heal ourselves the natural way.

Synthetic medication is unnatural because, although the ingredients were originally pure, they have become warped and altered to create a chemical that is used to treat symptoms and ailments. When you take these medications, as stated earlier, you are not allowing your body to restore itself. It quits working on the problem because you have allowed a foreign substance to do the job for you. *Natural supplements encourage the body to restore any imbalance so it can function on its own.* This is the *exact* reason I wanted to find a natural source to treat PCOS; I wanted my body, after several months or even a few years, to be able to operate efficiently and optimally on its own. I didn't mind taking supplements as long as it was a means to an end; something that I could eventually quit taking, that didn't harm my body or cause it to malfunction.

Birth control, blood sugar medication, anti-androgens, acne prescriptions, and fertility drugs all come with side effects, and your body likely cannot function without them. If you are taking or have taken any of these, I am not judging, just informing. I have taken many prescription and over-the-counter drugs in my life. You know, deep down, that this is not the way your body was intended to operate. I have never, ever known any woman who takes a multitude of prescription medication to be truly healthy. I had a client once who was only in her late thirties and taking a ton of different medications. She took so many pills that, to keep track of the names, she had to keep the list in her purse. Despite her many efforts, this woman could not lose the excess weight she carried, no matter how much she exercised and ate right. I tried to explain to her that her body would not give her true health until she freed it from so many medications. Of course, I would never recommend you stop taking any medication without first consulting your doctor, but she wouldn't even consider treating herself naturally. She, like so many others, was under the assumption that she "can't make it without her pills."

In *Master Your Metabolism*, Jillian Michaels reports that a major review concluded that many classes of pharmaceutical medications contribute to weight gain (including **antidiabetics**, antihistamines, **contraceptives**, steroid hormones and psychotropics like antipsychotics, antidepressants and mood stabilizers). She further points out that, "Because our medical system doesn't think holistically, your doctor could prescribe one drug to help you achieve the desired results in one part of your system, while over in another, you're throwing a hormone level totally out of whack."[8]

Author of *Natural Cures "They" Don't Want You to Know About*, Kevin Trudeau says it this way:

"Think about this: Animals do not exercise and have

no obesity or weight problems...Chimpanzees and gorillas are great examples. They don't lose their teeth, they don't have arthritis, they don't have diabetes, they don't need insulin shots, they don't have cancer, they don't have asthma, they don't have allergies, they are not constipated, they don't have insomnia, and they live to be an equivalent of about 180 years old. Interestingly enough, they go through their entire lives without taking any prescription or nonprescription drugs."[9]

Of course, there are many different circumstances as to why someone is taking medication. I understand that there are some life-threatening diseases that may require medical help and pharmaceuticals. PCOS and insulin resistance *will become* life-threatening conditions if not controlled naturally. I urge you to take care of your body and health now and do it in the most holistic way so you don't manifest potentially serious illnesses.

Well-made and responsibly developed natural supplements do not come with side effects associated with pharmaceuticals. When taken properly, and, as instructed (by talking to your doctor first), supplements either do their job or not. When they are created with integrity and made with ingredients close to their original state as possible, holistic supplements can help the body do what it was meant to do: keep you healthy, whole and thriving.

When researching PCOS, I discovered a company whose PCOS protocol included supplements that were specifically formulated to address PCOS and insulin resistance. The nutraceuticals element to their PCOS System targeted the root cause of PCOS, thought to be insulin resistance, to help women reverse symptoms and take control over these conditions. The company, Insulite Laboratories, is comprised of a team of doctors and nutritional and exercise experts who want to provide women a natural option to synthetic birth control pills and insulin-regulating pills. They are a small company based out of Colorado in the United States, and also have Systems, including supplements, for pre-diabetes, metabolic syndrome, excess weight and obesity and diabetes management.[10]

I found this company the same week that I decided that birth control pills, insulin-regulating pills and fertility drugs would not be options. I wanted to allow my body to naturally regulate and heal itself of the damage that had been done. My mother owns and operates an online supplement store and read over, researched and approved of the Insulite Labs' nutraceuticals ingredients. I respected her opinion because she happens to be a whiz at identifying supplements and their effects on the body. She has always taken the natural approach to combat any type of illness or imbalance.

What I love most about the Insulite System's nutraceuticals program is the fact that they combine an array of ingredients in each of the four PCOS formulas (listed in Appendix B). It would cost a fortune to take each of the vital nutrients in each pill if you bought them separately. It is the best investment you could ever make for your body, and it far outweighs the long-term medical costs associated with insurance, co-pays, and complications associated with diabetes, infertility and other problems that come with PCOS and insulin resistance. Furthermore, the emotional and psychological repercussions that come with being overweight, sick and tired year after year are far more costly to me than any monetary expenditure.

I look at supplements as an investment in my health. It is what many holistic practitioners and consumers call "preventative medicine." I have been taking supplements since August 2008, and within a short time I saw amazing changes. I was able to burn body fat and lose weight because the combination of ingredients specifically targeted my body's production of and response to insulin. My hormones were naturally balanced thus regulating my menstrual period and improving digestion. Over a long period of time, the supplements have helped women permanently lose weight, restore hormones and naturally get pregnant.[10]

I had such great results with Insulite Labs' nutraceuticals formulas that I now do voluntary coaching calls for them. I am a coach once a month and talk to women about the PCOS System and dealing with the condition.

It is obvious that I prefer Insulite Labs as a source for supplements to combat PCOS and insulin resistance. I have many women who love Insulite Labs, and others who want to try another company. You can do what you think is right. I am here to simply give you the facts of what worked for me in the shortest amount of time. If you wish to experiment with other brands, supplements or programs, go right ahead. I wrote this book so you could see exactly what I did. For those who do not want to try many different options to overcome

PCOS and simply want the shortcut, this is it.

I am now the Spokesperson for Insulite Labs because they have done wonders for me. I prefer them over others because I believe their program works. I would never recommend a company or product that I haven't personally used. There is more information regarding their program in the Appendix. However, I will discuss other supplements you can take if you do not want to use Insulite Labs. I do not wish to push any company or product on you. *I want you to do your due diligence and find a program that works for you.* There are other companies that have good products for women with PCOS. Look around, do some research and find what works for you.

If you do not want to, do not have access to, or cannot afford to go on a company's supplement program, there are other supplements you can take. I recommend you take four basic supplements that may help ease the symptoms of PCOS and insulin resistance. If I were you, I would take a really great **multivitamin**, containing all of the vitamins, mineral and nutrients you need on a daily basis, along with **Chromium**, **Evening Primrose Oil** and a **Probiotic** tablet or powder. There a few really great multivitamins, and I recommend New Chapter's Every Woman's One Daily and Pure Essence Labs' One n' Only Women's Formula. When a multivitamin is organic or pharmaceutical grade, you can *feel* the difference as opposed to a generic multivitamin. These multi's are great because they fill in the nutritional gaps from not having a healthy, balanced diet.

Chromium Picolinate (I took around 500mcg daily) helps to increase the cells' sensitivity to insulin, thereby increasing your body's response to insulin. Women with insulin resistance experience resistance to the blood glucose and insulin being produced. When glucose and insulin are not being properly used, you will easily store fat. Excess insulin also causes havoc with hormones, and it can damage the lining of our blood vessels thereby causing cardiovascular issues. Chromium helps to increase sensitivity to insulin.

Evening Primrose Oil, in my opinion, is a miracle pill. I used to take it every day before the nutraceuticals program, and I still occasionally take it if I need a "mood boost." Evening Primrose Oil is perfect for hormonal balance and it has been known to decrease symptoms like irritability, cramps, hot flashes, night sweats, headaches and muscular pain associated with PMS and menopause. I really like Barlean's Organic Oils, but you can use whichever company you prefer. If you suffer from serious hormonal imbalance, one to two pills a day should work for you. Otherwise, take one pill a day until you feel relief, then take one pill every other day and so on.

A really great Probiotic in the form of a pill or powder (I prefer powder) can aid in digestion, improve immunity and curb sugar and carbohydrate cravings. It does these things because it puts more "good bacteria" back in the body and regulates the digestive systems in the body. When digestion is under control and functioning properly, you have more energy, fewer cravings, less bloating, and improved health.

These supplemental options are your choice; I just wanted to give you a recommendation of what I would take if I chose not to take part in the comprehensive nutraceuticals program.

The reason I made this the 3rd step in the "Triple Threat" approach to overcome PCOS is because it will be easier to see results from steps 1 and 2 once you are filling your body with wholesome nutrients. Not to mention, a good combination of supplements will help you tackle healthy eating described in step 2. When cravings and constant, insatiable hunger are not an issue, choosing, preparing and eating the right foods will be a breeze. The nutrition portion of this program is so much more easily accomplished when taking nutraceuticals.

I understand that it can be a tough commitment to afford supplements on a tight budget. When I started taking them, my husband and I had just married, and like most other young, married couples, we had a mortgage and bills and were essentially broke. I was working at a holistic retreat center at the time, making 10 dollars an hour, working a little more than part time. Trust me, I know what it means to be broke, poor and out of answers, but this was an "investment" we knew had to be made for the sake of my health, happiness and mental sanity.

Can you put a price on overcoming a condition? To us, it was priceless. We cut back on eating out and other unnecessary purchases to afford supplements. I wouldn't recommend this step if I didn't believe that you would absolutely benefit from it. My reputation is on the line, and I will *never* recommend something I have not personally tried myself. These supplements make up an entire "step" in my 3-step program; *yes, I believe it's that important.*

Taking supplements didn't just help me reverse my symptoms of PCOS and insulin resistance. My results inspired me to become a personal trainer and life coach for women, start my own company, work from home full-time, and write, record and publish many information products to help other women around the globe. Being a part of an effective supplement program helped me gain clarity as to who I am and what my place is in this world. They did so much more than bringing back my menstrual period and helping me shed weight. Conquering my condition helped me focus my time, money and energy on more serious, important matters in my life. It's time you started focusing on who it is you want to be, and it starts right now as you decide whether or not your health is worth it.

Let's Sum It Up:

- Exercise and eating right only may not help control or overcome PCOS and insulin resistance.
- Taking "synthetic" medications to control PCOS and insulin resistance is costly and can be detrimental to your long-term health.
- Do some research and find a supplement program for women with PCOS and insulin resistance.
- If you don't want to or can't afford a supplement program, take a great multivitamin, Chromium, Evening Primrose Oil and a Probiotic. These four supplements can be very helpful in reducing the symptoms of both conditions.
- Your health is an investment. You have to decide whether or not your body is worth it.

Chapter 18

Putting it into Action

Congratulations on making it through the 3-step, "Triple Threat" approach! By reading this far, you have already proven that you are serious about proactively changing your life. If you are feeling a bit overwhelmed, please know that you do not have to take on all 3 steps at once. You don't have to be perfect, and you certainly don't have to give up your eating habits tomorrow. You must, however, begin to make some small changes. Some of you will have to make more changes than others, but after a while, your efforts will snowball and you will be amazed at the progress you make.

When I first started studying nutrition in 2002, I was eating a consistent diet of hotdogs, fried foods and ice cream. Instead of going crazy and throwing everything out of my cupboards, I looked at everything I was eating and made a small healthy switch every week. If I was already eating a turkey sandwich with cheese on white bread, I switched to whole wheat bread and cut the piece of cheese in half. If I was used to eating fried chicken, I would opt for the grilled chicken. I substituted baked beans for fries. Instead of cereal, I ate oatmeal with honey and milk. I even made the switch from drinking whole milk to almond milk. Yum!

Notice how I did not make gargantuan, life-altering food changes in one day. I simply looked at what I already liked to eat and creatively thought of a healthier substitution. Some women have an exotic palate; sometimes they eat in a way that stems from their particular culture. A friend told me she ate pork and rice at every family get together. "How can I eat healthier? It's impossible," she would tell me. I told her to be the daredevil guest who brings black beans and *brown* rice along with marinated, slow cooked *chicken* instead of pork. Yes, it might upset her family, but she was willing to make the change because her body and health condition were more frustrating and heartbreaking than the complaints from her family.

When you make healthy changes, some family members may initially get upset, but in the end it's about what kind of body, health and life you want. I love to bring my own desserts and side dishes to parties and family holiday gatherings because it ensures that I will have something healthy and delicious to eat. No offense to my wonderful relatives, but some of them are known for their less-than-healthy dishes, and it's not always good for my waistline. The bottom line is that your health should be your number one priority.

By combining my Triple Threat, 3-step approach, you will look better, feel better and essentially reverse many of your symptoms associated with Polycystic Ovarian Syndrome and insulin resistance. Now I will ask, "What will your life be like when you have beautiful skin; regulated (or more normalized) menstrual periods without PMS; fewer cravings, more energy and natural weight loss?" Can you imagine a life like this? I want you to get excited because by using my tried-and-proved exercise, nutrition and supplement program, you will see results like these!

4 Week Plan

I know you have taken in a lot of information in this book, so I want to leave you with a plan that will help you implement changes in your current lifestyle over the next 4 weeks. It may seem difficult in the beginning, but just remember that as your health improves, it will all be worth it. After all, I did it the long, challenging way, so this should be much simpler for you. Learn from my mistakes and make it as easy as possible on yourself. Let me know if I can help out at all, and I look forward to hearing about your changes.

Week 1: *Sit down and map out how you want these next 4 weeks to go down.* Which step will you tackle first? Do you want to follow my instructions, step by step, implementing exercise, nutrition and nutraceuticals? Write down what you will start doing with exercise, taking supplements, and nutrition. Join a gym, purchase exercise equipment for your home or recruit an exercise buddy. Start planning healthy meals with a protein and carbohydrate. Research Insulite Labs' nutraceuticals or another supplement company that works for you.

If you're doing exercise first, map out the days you will do steady-state cardio, intervals and strength training (example plan in Appendix B). I suggest you begin implementing 1 day of each type of exercise in the first two weeks, and add in 1 additional day of exercises every week thereafter. For instance, week 1, you will do some form of all three types of exercises (steady-state, intervals and strength training), and week 2, you can add 1 day to steady-state. In week 3, cut back on steady-state and add 1 day of intervals. Week 4, add in 1 day of strength training

Week 2: *Start designing your meal plan.* You can use the meal plan template in Appendix B to create daily and weekly meal plans. Experiment with grocery shopping and try cooking different meals. I don't like to cook a lot of fancy things, but I definitely get creative with my meals. For instance, if you want chicken, a sweet potato and some vegetables for dinner, why not "crust" the chicken with grated sweet potatoes, grill it in a pan, and roast some vegetables with 2 tablespoons of Olive Oil? Doesn't that sound delicious? I gave you food charts in the Appendix so you could get the "idea" of eating whole foods and combining a protein and carbohydrate with a few good fats. However, you don't have to limit yourself and eat boring stuff all day. Get inventive with your meals: you'll look forward to preparing *and* eating them!

Week 3: *Research supplements.* Search around for a program that might work for you, or find at least one individual supplement you want to try. I highly recommend the nutraceuticals in Insulite Labs' PCOS System, as mentioned in Step 3 of my "Triple Threat" approach to combat PCOS; but you need to decide what's right for you. You can find more information on the nutraceuticals in the Insulite PCOS System in Appendix B. No matter what, make a decision and do your due diligence on what you put in your body.

Week 4: *Begin making time in your daily schedule for self-care.* I wrote this book so I could give you the essential information or what I call the "outer tools" to overcoming PCOS, but the truth is that it all begins with your mindset. If you are not actively making time to take care of yourself and plant positivity, joy and love in your life, negative "weeds" such as fear, resentment and worthlessness will grow instead. The only reason I and the women I coach are as motivated, energetic and successful as we are is because we take time daily to create a space of gratitude and love, so we are more likely to exercise, nourish our bodies with whole foods and supplement with vitamins. Succeeding in anything takes time, so you must create a constant state of appreciation, warmth and love RIGHT NOW. This comes by consistently taking time in your daily schedule to read inspirational quotes, scripture or books, praying and meditating, and writing or speaking things you are grateful for. I have the women I coach take at least 15 minutes every single morning to do this, and I personally take 60 minutes of "personal time" every day to create this abundant space. Because of this daily ritual, I am happier, healthier, and more resilient to obstacles that used to hold me back. I promise, even if it takes months to see good results in your efforts to overcome PCOS, by taking time for yourself, you will instantly feel more alive and love the life you live. Managing your thoughts and emotions has so much power, and making a commitment to yourself to do this morning ritual will give you control over these things. Take time, right now, and schedule 15 minutes for yourself tomorrow morning. Wake up earlier if you have to, and write down what you will do to start off the day with gratitude, love and excitement! You will see just how amazing this small task makes you feel.

Go Forth!

I'm so proud of you for making it this far and choosing to believe that you can overcome PCOS! I know you are going to see great results. Just remember to keep fighting and pushing until you get to where you want to be. Whether you have 30 pounds to lose or 300, the tools you have learned in this book will give you the results you want. The bottom line is to persist until you succeed. And don't forget: EVERYTHING begins with your mental attitude. Whatever you have read in this book, as simple as may have sounded, your mindset will determine your outcome. So, be sure to work on you and the rest will fall into place. Never, ever give up. As my mentor says, "Unsuccessful people do what is comfortable and convenient. Successful people do whatever it takes!" Go over that statement with me again: To be successful, we must do WHATEVER IT TAKES. I know you can do this. It's up to you to keep other women with PCOS and insulin resistance inspired to make changes. Your results will help so many other women feel freedom from these conditions. I believe in you, and I wish you love and all the happiness in the world.

Appendix A

Creating Healthy Meal Plans

Choose from the lists below and create 4 to 5 daily meals using a protein and carbohydrate. Be sure to use "good" fats in some meals. I have provided you with the appropriate portion sizes for most foods, as well as a "meal planner" so you can track your meals. Below you will also find a sample meal plan of some of my typical meals. Have fun!

Protein Chart

Protein Choices	Serving Sizes
Lean red meat, Poultry or Fish	3 – 5 oz.
Tofu or Tempeh	80 – 160 grams
Eggs or Egg Whites	1 Whole Egg & 1 – 2 Egg Whites; 2 -3 Egg Whites
Beans or Legumes	½ cup
Yogurt	1 cup
Nuts	2 oz or 2 TBS

Carbohydrate Chart

Carbohydrate: Grains	Serv. Size
100% Brown Rice, Whole Grain, Wheat, Spelt, or Sprouted Grain Products (Cereals or Pastas)	½ cup
Bread Products (bagels, bread, English muffin)	1 slice
Oatmeal (either slow-cooking or rolled oats)	½ cup
Brown Rice, Quinoa, Whole Grain Couscous, Amaranth, Barley	½ cup

Carbohydrates: Unlimited Vegetables and Fruits		
Apples	Cucumbers	Onions and Garlic
Mushrooms	Romaine	Spinach and Kale
Kiwis	Blueberries	Raspberries
Peppers	Broccoli	Green Beans
Celery	Strawberries	Tomatoes

Carbohydrates: Small Portions of Vegetables and Fruits		
Banana (1 small)	Cantaloupe (2 slices)	Melons (2 slices)
Grapes (1 – 2 cups)	Oranges (1 whole)	Grapefruit (1/2)
Squash (1 cup)	Cauliflower (1 cup)	Mango (1 small)
Dried Fruit (1/2 cup)	Peas/Pea Pods	Potatoes (4 oz.)
Carrots (1 cup)	Zucchini (1 cup)	Pineapple (1 cup)

For more carbohydrate info, check the Glycemic Index below.

Substitution Guide

Here is a quick and easy reference to making healthy substitutions to your favorite foods.

Instead of eating...	Try eating...
Pork	(Organic) Lean Red Meat or Poultry
Fried Foods	Grilled, Broiled, Steamed or Poached Foods
High Fructose Corn Syrup, Refined Sugar or Artificial Sweeteners	100% Maple Syrup, Agave, Honey, or Stevia
Refined flour (in bread, cereal, pasta, bagels, muffins, etc.)	100% Whole wheat, grain, spelt or sprouted grains (like in Ezekiel products), or brown rice flour
Milk	Almond, Hemp or Rice Milk
Lunch Meat	Organic deli meat (anything without preservatives)
Chips, Cookies, Crackers	Organic baked chips, cookies and crackers
Alcohol	Organic Red Wine
Protein Bar	Lara Bars

Glycemic Index

The Glycemic Index is a vast resource for finding your favorite foods and how they are rated according to their impact on your blood sugar levels. Since it is so comprehensive, I suggest you visit www.glycemicindex.com and search any particular food to find out which grains, vegetables and fruits are best to eat. Hint: The lower foods on the Glycemic Index have a positive effect on your body.

Clip out the meal planner below.

Meal	Meal Description	Alternative Meal
Notes:		

Sample Meal Plan: Katie Humphrey

Meal	Meal Description	Alternative Meal
Meal 1 (Breakfast)	Protein shake w/ Almond Milk, 1 banana and veggie protein mix	
Meal 2 (3 hours later)	2 oz. raw nuts and seeds	Lara Bar
Meal 3 (3 hours later)	Large salad with berries, ½ avocado, handful sliced almonds, and lime juice	Steamed veggies and black bean soup
Meal 4 (3 hours later)	1 grapefruit and some vegetable-laden soup	Hummus and crackers
Meal 5 (dinner)	4-5 oz. wild caught fish, brown rice and lots of steamed or roasted veggies	4-5 oz. wild caught fish over large salad with lemon juice
Meal 6 (not typical)	Apple with 2 TBS raw almonds	
Notes: Dessert (optional) might be organic dark chocolate or cut up pineapple.		

Sample Monthly Exercise Schedule

Day 1	Day2	Day 3	Day 4	Day 5	Day 6	Day7
Steady-state		Intervals			Strength training	
Steady-state		Intervals	Steady-state		Strength training	
Steady-state	Intervals		Strength training		Intervals	
Steady-state	Intervals	Strength training		Steady-state	Strength training	

Appendix B

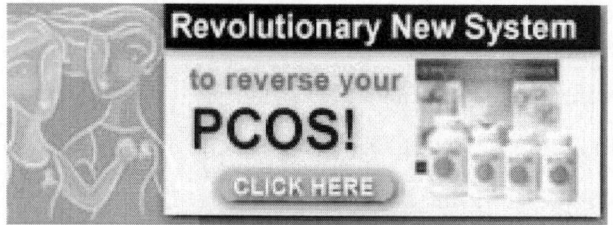
Insulite Laboratories is the company that supplies my nutraceuticals as a part of its PCOS System. I have been using them since August 2008. I have tried other companies for supplements and products that promise hormonal balance and leave me disappointed. I highly recommend Insulite Laboratories because they are the best at what they do, and they genuinely care about your personal well-being. If you would like more information to get started on their PCOS system, my affiliate link is www.PCOSSystem.com. They are based in the United States, but they ship internationally. They have a 90-day, 100% money-back guarantee.

    The nutraceuticals regimen consists of 4 different formulas. They are InsulX, RejuvenX, PCOS+, and GlucX. The InsulX and RejuvenX are taken together at 2 meals every day.[10] I take them at breakfast and lunch or at lunch and dinner. PCOS+ and GlucX are taken twice a day between meals. So I'm taking a combo of pills at one meal, a combo after the meal, a combo at the next meal, and the final combo after that meal. I have broken it down for you to give you an example of a typical day of taking these pills. You do not have to take them at or in between lunch and dinner; it is simply for the sake of showing you how you could do it.

This is how you could take the nutraceuticals:
- ✓   Lunch: InsulX and RejuenX
- ✓   1 hour after lunch: PCOS + and GlucX
- ✓   Dinner: InsulX and RejuvenX
- ✓   1 hour after dinner: PCOS + and GlucX

This sounds like a lot of pills to take. *Initially it was, but I was willing to do anything to lose weight and feel better.* To make it easier, I put the right combination of pills in 2 different sandwich bags and keep them in my purse. If I am on vacation or out to dinner, I can easily remember to take my pills. After a month or two, the pills are easy to take because it becomes a habit.

Like I mentioned before, these nutraceuticals have been created to contain all of the necessary ingredients you and I need to overcome PCOS and insulin resistance.

InsulX Ingredients*:

- **Vanadium (Sulfate)** - Restores blood glucose, lowers cholesterol, increases insulin sensitivity, improves glucose tolerance and metabolism, decreases body fat and reduces appetite naturally.

- **Chromium (GTF Niacinate)** - Supports insulin binding to cells and decreases cholesterol and insulin levels. Boosts insulin response to glucose.

- **Alpha Lipoic Acid** - Increases insulin sensitivity and lowers glucose levels. Provides antioxidant activity, scavenges free radicals, supports glucose transport and extends the functional capacity of Vitamin C, Vitamin E, and Co Q 10.

- **Magnesium (Amino Acid Chelate)** - Positively affects insulin secretion/action and improves cholesterol profile. (Lower than normal levels of Magnesium Glycinate are associated with Insulin Resistance, glucose intolerance and hyperinsulinemia.)

- **Zinc (Picolinate)** - Lowers insulin concentration and improves insulin sensitivity.

- **L-Carnitine (Tartrate)** - Improves insulin sensitivity.

- **Copper (Citrate)** - Balances zinc and supports its ability to lower insulin concentration.

- **Calcium (Citrate/Malate)** - Reduces fasting insulin levels, increases insulin sensitivity and regulates fat tissue.

- **Biotin USP** - Involved in the manufacture and release of insulin; a cofactor required for the synthesis and oxidation of fatty acids.

- **Manganese (Citrate)** - Reverses glucose intolerance, a deficiency associated with diabetes.

- **Pancreatic Tissue** - Contains specific amino acids in the correct proportions to supply growth, balance and repair factors of the pancreas.

- **Adrenal Tissue** - Contains specific amino acids to supply growth, balance and repair factors of the adrenals.
- **Protease and Amylase** - Improve absorption and digestion of proteins and nutrient absorption.

RejuvenX Ingredients*:

- **Vitamin C from calcium ascorbate** - Balances Vitamin C deficiency that induces disordered glucose regulation, improves glucose tolerance and scavenges free radicals. Reduces damage to arteries and arterioles and reduces glycosylation.
- **CoQ10 (Ubiquinone)** - Lowers glucose and insulin levels and plays a major role in carbohydrate metabolism. Aids peripheral glucose utilization while lowering fasting blood sugar.
- **Vitamin B12 (Cyanocobalamin)** - Reduces neuropathy associated with diabetes, sorbitol accumulation, muscle weakness and tingling.
- **Folic Acid (Calcium Folinate)** - Ensures sufficient folate status to aid in the prevention of many chronic diseases (e.g. atherosclerosis, anemia, heart disease) and reverses homocysteine levels.
- **Quercitin** - Contains antioxidant, anticarcinogenic and anti-inflammatory properties to inhibit free radical production. Reduces intracellular accumulation of sorbitol that is implicated in the pathogenesis of cataracts, retinopathies, neuropathies and other disorders.

- **Bilberry Extract** - Improves microcirculation and protects the vessels of the eyes in particular with potent antioxidants.

- **Grape Seed Extract** - Reduces free radicals and possesses vital antibacterial, antiviral, anticarcinogenic, anti-inflammatory and anti-allergic effects. (Its antioxidant properties are 20 to 50 times stronger than Vitamins C and E.) Lowers cholesterol levels and prevents damage to the artery from elevated glucose and insulin levels.

- **Thiamin** - Thiamin (Vitamin B1) (as thiamin hcl) May help convert carbohydrates into energy. Thiamin is important for several bodily functions of the heart, muscles, and the nervous system.

- **Vitamin D** - Vitamin D (as cholecalciferol) Vitamin D plays a role in bone health and has an important role in immunity, wound healing, and hypertension. Vitamin D may also be known to affect insulin secretion and glucose tolerance in Type 2 diabetes.

- **Cinnamon Extract** - A recent controlled trial (1), comparing a placebo against cinnamon, demonstrated that doses of cassia cinnamomum—ranging from 1-6 grams a day provided in divided daily doses—produced some significant reductions in blood sugar levels, total cholesterol levels, triglyceride levels and finally even lower levels of LDL lipoproteins. RejuvenX provides 1.2 grams cinnamon per dose.

PCOS+ Ingredients*:

- **Saw Palmetto (berries)** - a 5-alpha reductase inhibitor impedes testosterone conversion and reduces circulating testosterone (androgens).
- **Vitex Agnus Castus (Chaste tree berry)** - Improves menstrual regularity, supports luteal phase of menstrual cycle and addresses hyperprolactinemia.
- **Stinging Nettle (root)** - Increases sex hormone-binding globulin.
- **Flax Seed** - Supports estrogen metabolism, which increases the production of protective estrogen metabolites and increases sex hormone-binding globulin.
- **Milk Thistle (seed, powdered extract)** - Supports liver function (phase 1 detoxification).

GlucX Ingredients*:

- **Guar Gum** - Decreases cholesterol, triglycerides and systolic blood pressure. Increases insulin sensitivity and regulates appetite.
- **Apple Pectin & Beet Powder** - Slows the absorption of glucose into the blood stream which reduces insulin response.
- **Fenugreek** - Reduces blood sugar and insulin following a meal, lowers cholesterol levels (LDL, TG and total Cholesterol), increases HDL and improves insulin response and glucose tolerance.

- **Milk Thistle** - Diminishes fasting blood glucose, mean daily glucose and fasting insulin levels.

The combination of nutraceuticals will help to improve glucose and insulin response, regulate and balance estrogen and testosterone levels, and possibly reduce blood cholesterol, high blood pressure and triglyceride levels. They are designed to give you relief to symptoms like weight gain, fatigue, acne, mood swings, facial and body hair, and poor metabolism, as well as long-term care to help thwart infertility, diabetes, and problems associated with obesity.[10]

The plan offers a 90 day risk-free 100% guarantee if it doesn't work for you. You cannot lose on this program, and I bet you see results sooner than 6 months. However, most doctors agree that to see viable results from any type of pill, you should take it for at least 3 months. I recommend taking the nutraceuticals for at least 6 months if you want to see serious changes. Think of it this way; it took how many years to come to this place with PCOS and insulin resistance? What is another 6 months, especially if it means you could change your condition? To me, 6 months was nothing, and I wouldn't have cared if it took a year; I am so grateful that I found something that helped me. Here is the link, again, to get started on the Insulite PCOS System: www.PCOSSystem.com.

Additional PCOS Treatment Options

Acupuncture is a highly recommended therapy as a natural way to balance hormones and restore a regular menses. I have heard many naturopathic doctors recommend acupuncture, and I even read a magazine article recently that said: "One-Word Answer," and below was, "Acupuncture: The practice can help treat polycystic ovary syndrome (PCOS), a condition that can lead to irregular menstrual periods and infertility. Acupuncture reduces harmful levels of nerve activity caused by PCOS and increases the likelihood of regular monthly cycles." The information source was the American Journal of Physiology – Regulatory, Integrative and Comparative Physiology.

Yoga is a fantastic way to reduce stress and increase energy and the mind-body connection. You become more flexible and elongated, and it's an essential part to being healthy and in great shape.

Recommended Reading

For your hormonal health:
The Eat Clean Diet by Tosca Reno
Master Your Metabolism by Jillian Michaels
Skinny Bitch by Kim Barnouin and Rory Freedman

For creating a positive mental attitude:
Awaken the Giant Within by Anthony Robbins
Think and Grow Rich by Napoleon Hill
The Seven Spiritual Laws of Success by Deepak Chopra
The Greatest Salesman in the World by Og Mandino

Notes

1. United States of America. U.S. Department of Health and Human Services. The National Women's Health Information Center. *Polycystic Ovarian Syndrome (PCOS)*. Web. <http://www.womenshealth.gov/faq/polycystic-ovary-syndrome.cfm>.

2. "Long Term Complications of Diabetes." *Merck*. The Merck Manual of Health and Aging. Web. <http://www.merck.com/pubs/mmanual_ha/tables/tb34_1.html>.

3. Reid, Edward. *Exercise and insulin* (2009). *Www.faq.org*. Advameg, Inc., 22 Oct. 2009. Web. <http://www.faqs.org/faqs/diabetes/faq/part1/section-15.html>.

4. Physical Activity (2009). Healthy Places. Centers for Disease Control and Prevention. Web. <http://www.cdc.gov/HEALTHYPLACES/healthtopics/physactivity.htm>.

5. Academy, National. *NASM Essentials of Personal Fitness Training*. 3rd ed. Philadelphia: Lippincott Williams & Wilkins, 2007. Print.

6. "Fast Facts on Osteoporosis." *NOF - Bone Mass Measurement*. National Osteoporosis Foundation. Web. <http://www.nof.org/osteoporosis/diseasefacts.htm>.

7. Leggatt/Muscle & Fitness/Hers, Jaime. "FAQS: training over 40; What 40-somethings should know about diet, exercise and

metabolism." *FAQS: training over 40; What 40-somethings should know about diet, exercise and metabolism* (2003). *Www.Findarticles.com.* BNET, Apr. 2003. Web. <http://findarticles.com/p/articles/mi_m0KGB/is_3_4/ai_n6003004/>.

8. Michaels, Jillian, and Mariska Van Aalst. *Master Your Metabolism.* New York: Crown, 2009. Print.

9. Trudeau, Kevin. *Natural Cures "They" Don't Want You To Know About.* Grand Rapids: Alliance, 2005. Print.

10. Insulite Laboratories | Reversing Insulin Resistance. Web. 09 Feb. 2010. <http://www.insulitelabs.com>.

11. Reno, Tosca. *The Eat-Clean Diet Fast Fat-Loss that lasts Forever!* Grand Rapids: Robert Kennedy, 2007. Print.

12. *Control Your Cravings.* Men's Health. Web. <http://www.menshealth.com/men/nutrition/diet-strategies/blood-sugar/article/a3478c7f2eb40110VgnVCM20000012281eac>.

13. Davis, Jeanie L. Lose Weight: Eat Breakfast: 1-3. Healthy Eating & Diet. WebMD. Web. <http://www.webmd.com/diet/features/lose-weight-eat-breakfast>.

14. Austin, Denise, and Amy Campbell. Eat Carbs, Lose Weight Drop All the Pounds You Want without Giving Up the Foods You Love. New York: Rodale, 2005. Print.

15. *The Glycemic Index.* Web. 09 Feb. 2010. <http://www.glycemicindex.com>.

16. Barnouin, Kim, and Rory Freedman. *Skinny Bitch.* New York: Running Book, 2005. Print.

17. Colbert, Don. Toxic Relief Restore Health and Energy Through Fasting and Detoxification. New York: Siloam, 2003. Print.

About the Author

As a woman who struggled for years with the devastating side effects of PCOS, insulin resistance and hypoglycemia, Katie Humphrey learned effective ways to address these conditions and see positive, long-lasting results. Katie now empowers both women and girls with PCOS to produce extraordinary results in their health and other areas of life by managing their mental and emotional wellbeing.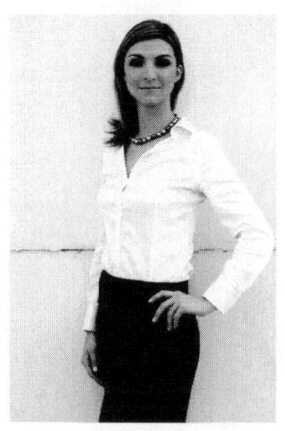

Katie is a motivational speaker, author, and international health coach and holds a B.A. in Business Administration from Stetson University. She is an NASM Certified Personal Trainer, author of *Freedom from PCOS* and Spokesperson for PCOS Insulite Laboratories.

Katie has been featured in Shape.com, ChickRx, the PCOSA and has been interviewed on dozens of national radio shows.

Katie empowers women through private coaching, group coaching, live events and private retreats.

Katie is owner of JK Humphrey International and resides in Ocala, Florida with her husband.

Printed in Great Britain
by Amazon.co.uk, Ltd.,
Marston Gate.